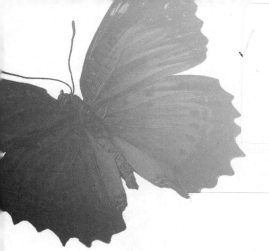

Expanding Nursing and Health Care Practice

Series Editor: Lynne Wigens

Optimising Learning through Practice

Lynne Wigens

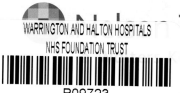

Nelson Thornes

luwer business

Published in 2006 by:
Nelson Thornes Ltd
Delta Place
27 Bath Road
CHELTENHAM
GL53 7TH
United Kingdom

06 07 08 09 10 / 10 9 8 7 6 5 4 3 2 1

A catalogue record for this book is available from the British Library

ISBN 0–7487–8365–2

Cover photograph by Stockbyte RF (NT)
Illustrations by Florence Production Ltd, Stoodleigh, Devon
Page make-up by Florence Production Ltd, Stoodleigh, Devon

Printed by UniPrint Hungary Kft, Székesfehérvár

Contents

Acknowledgements

I would like to thank the following people:

Paul, Matthew and Samuel Wigens, for all their support and encouragement.

Health professional students, and colleagues, for their comments which have informed much of this text.

Lisa Fraley and Helen Broadfield of Nelson Thornes for all their help and support throughout the inception and development of this book, and its associated series.

I would also like to remember Dr Terry Phillips who provided me with thoughtful and dedicated academic supervision for my doctoral thesis, which was the initial springboard for this book.

Preface

Health care professionals learn constantly through their practice. This book aims to provide newly qualified health professionals, mentors and students with the background, theory and practical knowledge to get the most out of practice and to harness all forms of learning opportunity. My interest in learning through practice is based on many years of working and teaching within education and service settings, as a Senior Lecturer and over the past few years as an Assistant Director of Nursing.

The book is divided into chapters covering key areas. In each chapter the subject is considered from the stance of a student as well as that of a qualified health care professional (mentors, practice teachers, preceptors, clinical supervisors and practice educators), using theoretical and practical examples. Each chapter starts with some **Learning outcomes** to signpost the main aspects covered within the chapter and incorporates a range of features to help you to assess your understanding and engage actively with the content being explored. Important educational words are defined under **Keywords** in the margin. When a section in a chapter has covered a range of complex content, this is summarised in a **Key points** feature. You are given opportunities to expand your learning through **Over to you**, **Case study**, **Clinical Caseload**, **Reflective** and **Evidence base activities**, which are interspersed throughout the book. I have also included a **Health professional speaks** feature in which a health care professional talks about practical situations and caseload management issues. **Rapid recap** questions at the end of each chapter give the reader a chance to assess what they have learnt from reading the text.

What makes this book different from many other texts is that it looks at individual and social learning, which, I believe, are inextricably linked. The book is, therefore, context related, focuses on the practical appreciation of learning theories, and covers the principles of sound mentorship and clinical supervision. This book incorporates recent evidence regarding situated learning, the NHS knowledge and skills framework and the influence of learning communities on the health care practice of students and qualified staff, and suggests the components that come together to make a 'good' clinical learning environment. Whether you are a student or an experienced practitioner, this book should offer insights to improve your own learning and your contribution to the learning of others, and may even be transformative in the way that you think about practice-based learning. As Heraclitus the Greek Philosopher (540–475BC) indicates:

> You can not step into the same river twice.

Not only is the context constantly changing, you also continually transform as you act and learn.

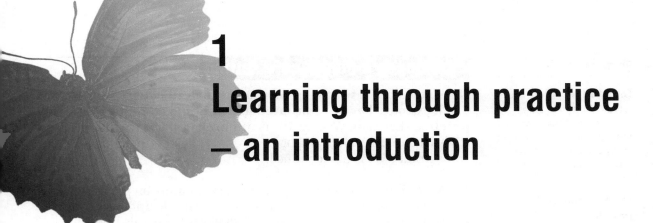

1
Learning through practice – an introduction

Learning outcomes

By the end of this chapter you should be able to:

★ Understand the overall structure and content of this book

★ Start to understand the concept of learning through practice

★ Recognise how this book has relevance to yourself as a learner and to your support of others in clinical settings

★ Appreciate how important learning through practice is in bridging the theory and practice 'gap'.

Introduction

In this book you will examine learning through practice, what it is and why it is important, not only for your own learning and for the development of your professional practice but also for supporting others in their clinical learning. The purpose of this introductory chapter is to set the scene. You can then approach the rest of the book with an understanding of what you are trying to achieve in developing your learning from your practice experiences. I have also used this section to introduce the rest of the book to you.

The book covers a range of issues, theories and practical examples regarding learning through practice and is a helpful resource for students who want to get the most from their clinical placements and for mentors and supervisors who facilitate learning within clinical settings. Using evidence and research throughout, the book demonstrates the practical application of situated learning and learning communities within health care education and offers a range of interactive exercises and case studies.

The following aspects of learning through practice are examined:

- making the best of use of clinical learning opportunities
- identifying individual learning needs, i.e. learning contracts and personal development plans
- clinical supervision, mentorship and preceptorship
- problem-based and action learning
- evidencing practice learning, i.e. portfolios, competencies, assessment and evaluation
- the adult learner and lifelong learning
- improving the learning environment and managing constraints
- the wider context of continuous professional development, including training needs analysis and practice educator roles.

Keywords

Situated learning

Situated learning takes place in the setting where the learning will be applied, and assumes that social processes will affect this learning

Communities of practice

Learning is seen as an act of membership and participation in a community of practice, which is the social group that integrates knowledge and situated learning into its life and working

Learning in a health care setting

One of the ways in which this book differs from other texts available is that it explores the role of **situated learning** and **communities of practice** (Lave and Wenger, 1991) within clinical practice, using case study data to aid understanding.

As Eraut (1994) has identified:

> Apart from the limited though valuable literature on professional socialisation, we know very little about what is learnt during the period of initial qualification . . . Still less is known about the subsequent learning, how and why professionals learn to apply, disregard or modify their initial training immediately after qualification, and to what extent continuing on-the-job learning contributes to their professional maturation, updating, promotion or reorientation.
>
> (Eraut, 1994, p. 40)

Within this book, some of Eraut's (1994) concerns – illustrated in the previous quote – will begin to be addressed. In order to get the most from learning through practice it is necessary to appreciate the complexity of learning within a health care setting. Take a look at the following case study, in which a registered nurse is observed going about her work on a hospital ward.

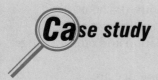
Case study

Prioritising work in a practice setting

A nurse was walking at a fast pace to get behind the nurses' station. During the first 10 minutes on the ward, I observed that she made decisions about the following:

1   She decided to telephone the police because a patient had died and she had been unable to contact the next of kin; she made the call.

2   She listened to a doctor's request for her to take out a venflon from a patient, as this was no longer in the right place (tissued), and to do a sitting and standing blood pressure recording to look for postural hypotension with another patient. Although acknowledging the request, she did not fulfil it during the 10-minute period.

3   She spoke in a welcoming way to a patient who was being transferred on his bed from the High Dependency Unit (HDU), following bowel surgery. The nurse noted that the patient's documentation was not suitable for this particular ward and so she took a few core care plans over to the patient and said, 'I'll catch up on the paperwork later'.

4   She walked around to a whiteboard that had all the patients' names on it and said to the student nurse working with her, 'Some of this care can be done this afternoon, because we won't have time this morning – like the removal of the epidural and the CVP (central venous pressure) line on the HDU transfer'.

How do you think this registered nurse had learnt to set priorities for the work that she had to do during the 10-minute period of the observation?

From reading this observational account, it starts to become clear that health care practitioners have to learn to meet many requirements at the same time. Indeed, the greatest nursing competence could be the ability to manage multiple demands. The nurse in the case study may have been surprised if you had asked her how she 'learnt' to deal with these demands, but one thing is pretty certain: she is unlikely to say that this was how she was taught during her nursing education. A student practitioner watching a qualified member of staff may find it difficult to grasp the 'knowledge' that underpins their work, particularly as every interpretation involves a point of view. As a practitioner goes about their professional work, their use of knowledge and their own knowledge creation cannot easily be separated because the use of an idea in a new context is itself a minor act of knowledge creation.

Health care practitioners perceive, experience, and learn to manage everyday practice in contexts where many things happen at the same time. As the record of the short observation given in the previous case study illustrates, it would be impractical to halt nursing practice to examine critically the processes in which nurses engage and through which they are learning to manage practice. Therefore, many nurse educators would argue that, for nurses to develop advanced understanding of the processes that they employ on a daily basis, they must develop the habit of regular critical reflection on practice (Jasper *et al.*, 2000; Johns and Freshwater, 1998). Paradoxically, as the observational excerpt shows, time for such reflection in practice is constrained by the need to act 'now', and a nurse soon develops a foundation of **tacit knowledge** to use in her daily tasks. Consequently, nursing learning remains largely implicit, and part of the task of this book is to help you to engage with and get the most from your practice and that of others.

Keywords

Tacit knowledge

The knowledge that people carry in their minds from their experience that they may not be aware of. It is seen as valuable to others as it is rooted in context, people, places, ideas and experiences. (Michael Polanyi (1951) originated this concept)

Using this book

In this book, I wish to reinforce the approach that learning is not a passive exercise and that the most effective way to learn from the written material is for you to interact with what you are reading. This is accomplished in a number of ways, particularly by considering the text in the light of your own experiences.

Each chapter commences by identifying the key elements that you will learn about in the text and contains activities that illustrate the issues with which the chapter deals. Through engagement with these activities you will see how the ideas presented translate into your own and other people's experiences. One example of this will be a 'reflective activity' that gives you time to reflect on the ideas that you are meeting and relate them in some way to your own experiences. As a result, you will be acquiring and consolidating the skills for learning through practice as you progress through the book. Throughout the book, you will meet new terms, ideas and words, which will be identified and explained. So that the use of educational terminology does not impede understanding, 'key words' will be defined in the margin, to help you to 'translate' the words for your own use and become comfortable with using the words and the concepts that they incorporate. A few 'rapid recap' questions are offered at the end of each chapter to allow you an opportunity to examine 'what you have learnt'.

It is impossible for any writer to construct a text that forces the reader to read it in one way and in one way only. Texts are sites of negotiation (Clark and Ivanic, 1997). The best I can do, as author, is to signpost readers through its formal structure. The book can be read in the following chapter sequencing, or you can choose to 'dip' into the sections that have most relevance to you at the time.

Chapter 2 looks at the 'adult learner' and higher education perspectives on learning. Whether you are reading this book as a student practitioner or a clinical supervisor, it is important to appreciate the educational theories that support educational programmes and practice learning. The differences between behaviourist, cognitive and humanistic approaches to learning are discussed, as well as the various forms of knowledge that can support learning through practice. Continuous professional development and lifelong learning have become increasingly important within health care and within this chapter these terms are examined in relation to individual and collective learning.

Most of your practice learning takes place within clinical placements or your clinical work setting, and the aspects that comprise 'good' clinical learning areas are examined within Chapter 3. The Quality Assurance Agency for Higher Education's code for practice placements (QAAHE, 2001) is looked at, and you are encouraged to consider your current clinical area. Ways of getting the most out of all clinical learning opportunities are discussed, and the chapter concludes by encouraging the evaluation of clinical placements.

All health care practitioners work in clinical teams, whether these are uni- or multiprofessional in nature, and the importance of these teams to learning through practice is explored in Chapter 4. The evidence base for situated learning and communities of practice is reviewed. Recognising the importance of professional identity and socialisation processes to learning to deliver health care will allow you to identify the effectiveness of your clinical team in supporting learning through practice.

Chapter 4 argues for the importance of clinical teams in practice-based learning, whereas Chapter 5 gives you the opportunity to reflect on individual learning and how your learning style can affect this. Being able to negotiate and construct learning contracts, learning outcomes, competencies and personal development plans is vital in optimising practice-based learning and tools for helping you to do this effectively are incorporated here within the book.

The importance of clinical educational roles to the learning environment is discussed in Chapter 6. Clinical supervisor, mentor, practice teacher and preceptor roles are defined; and crucial skills, such as assessing practice, role-modelling, encouraging reflection and skills development, and giving and receiving feedback, are looked at. Personal qualities and relationship development are also considered as these play a vital role in helping practitioners to make the transition from novice to expert.

Chapter 7 examines peer, problem-based and action learning, which has increasingly become the chosen approach for professional education. Understanding motivations to learn and the ways to get the most out of these methods is explored. Experiential learning is facilitated by the development of reflection, and guidance on how to develop reflective skills is given. The value of evidence-based practice and pragmatic approaches to action planning is also covered.

Even though learning through practice has been achieved, many practitioners find it difficult to provide evidence of this, whether to colleagues, mentors or to lecturers. It is a requirement of professional qualificatory courses to be assessed in practice, and evidence of this has to be retained for future reference. A qualified practitioner will need to keep a portfolio of their professional practice learning to show that they have kept their practice up to date. Chapter 8 outlines the range of evidence that can be offered to indicate learning through practice, including portfolios and profiles, critical incident analyses, career biographies, learning diaries, and documentation of competences and skills. Within this chapter, assessment from novice to expert practice levels is explored.

Understandably, everyday work in clinical settings has patient care as the priority, and this can be viewed as constraining learning through practice. Chapter 9 discusses possible barriers to work-based learning, such as high patient caseloads and professional agendas, and variations within clinical settings are examined. The concept of emotional labour is discussed, and ways to manage any constraints to learning through practice are offered for you to consider within your own clinical area.

Having looked at factors that may constrain learning through practice, the final chapter, Chapter 10, adopts a broader perspective. This chapter considers approaches that foster effective clinical learning environments and takes a step away from the clinical setting to explore the wider context of learning through practice at a national, local and organisational level. Curricular changes and academic-service partnership working is discussed. Changing curricula within health care – instigated at an educational institute level or by policy makers for education, training and development – can bring major challenges for learning through practice: one recent example of this is the mandated requirement for interprofessional learning within many qualificatory professional programmes. A systematic approach to education and training needs analysis is also discussed, and the role of practice educators and nurse teachers in supporting practice learning is explored.

The overall content of this book looks at learning as being both socially based and individualistic.

RRRRRRapid recap

Check your progress so far by working through each of the following questions.

1 What is situated learning?
2 What is a community of practice?
3 Define the term 'tacit knowledge'.
4 Give some examples of evidence that could be used within a professional portfolio.

If you have difficulty with one of these questions, read through the section again to refresh your understanding before moving on.

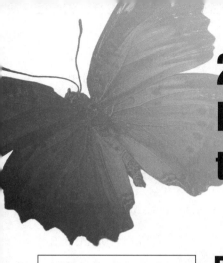

2
Linking educational theory to practice

Learning outcomes

By the end of this chapter you should be able to:

★ Explain adult and higher education perspectives on learning

★ Appreciate the differences between behaviourist, cognitive and humanistic theories of learning

★ Understand the importance of lifelong learning and continuous professional development to professional practice

★ Start to identify opportunities for learning within practice settings, and the different types of knowledge involved.

Introduction

In this chapter you will explore educational theories to aid understanding of learning through practice. Some educational issues are common to all health care professionals, such as adult and higher education perspectives on learning. In other ways, however, the health care setting is special in the way that this impacts on individual and collective learning.

We will consider a range of theories of learning broadly termed behaviourist, cognitive and humanistic and look at the importance of these to health care environments. The aim of the chapter is for you to understand and recognise how these educational theories help in appreciating different approaches to learning about practice.

Education theories for practice

Learning is something everyone does all of the time. There are two main stances on learning and the process of learning. It can be seen as either:

1 **Outcome based**: knowledge is taken in and absorbed by the learner and retained for future use; this is a building block approach, where knowledge is accumulated. Gagné (1985) took a systems view of learning, seeing information as being processed. The key elements involved in a systems way of looking at learning are the learner, the stimulus situation, the learner's memory, and their response to the situation. What is learnt may include intellectual skills, information, cognitive strategies, psychomotor skills, or attitudes.

> Learning is a change in human disposition or capability that persists over a period of time and is not simply ascribable to the process of growth.

> (Gagné, 1985, p. 2)

2 **Process based**: this entails a flexible network of ideas, knowledge and feelings, where learning involves a process of assembling, ordering or modifying understanding (termed 'assimilation' by Piaget, 1971). Learning as a process is grounded in experience, requiring resolution of conflicts between alternative ways of looking at and adapting to the world. It involves transactions between the learner and the environment and leads to the creation of knowledge.

> Learning is the process whereby knowledge is created through the transformation of experience.
>
> (Kolb, 1984a, p. 38)

The student's conception of what learning is, either as a product, a process, or both, can predict the quality of their learning (Marton and Saljo, 1984). The way that a learner views their learning affects whether learning is at a surface level or a deep level. It has been suggested that there are five main levels, with levels 1 to 3 perceived as 'surface' and levels 4 and 5 as 'deep' (Marton and Saljo, 1984).

Levels of learning

1   Learning is about increasing knowledge
2   Learning is about memorising and remembering
3   Learning is acquiring facts or skills to be used
4   Learning is about making sense and determining the meaning
5   Learning is about understanding reality

Learning that is deep and process based has perhaps been more influential within many professional education programmes. More recently, there has also been a movement to combine process and product within theories of learning. For instance, Jarvis (1995) combined both in the following 'meanings of learning':

- any more or less permanent change in behaviour which occurs as a result of practice
- a relatively permanent behavioural change as a result of experience
- the process whereby knowledge is created through the transformation of experience
- the process of transforming experience to knowledge, skills and attitudes
- memorising information.

Whether learning is meaningful is dependent on the learner's relationship to this new knowledge and their current cognitive working

(Pardoe, 2000). For this interpretation of learning to help resolve the outcome versus process debate, it is crucial to read Jarvis's (1995) meanings of learning from a stance that assumes that the terms 'experience' and 'practice' do not just refer to an individual but to the wider social context.

As well as understanding that individual factors affect learning, it is important to appreciate that the meaning of learning is not determined alone, but in conjunction with the experience of others in a socially and culturally agreed form (Lave and Wenger, 1991).

Educational theories

Apart from the product and process ways, there are three main approaches to understanding learning. In this section of the chapter, you will explore the behaviourist, cognitive and humanistic perspectives on learning and see how these may influence mentors and clinical supervisors in clinical settings.

Behaviourist learning theory

From a behaviourist stance, learning is the result of the application of consequences, that is, learners begin to connect certain responses with certain stimuli. According to behaviourism, there are two components to learning – Stimulus>Response. Different behavioural theories elaborate on this basic paradigm in different ways. Within the classical conditioning model, learning starts with an unconditioned response (a reflex) to an unconditioned (positive or negative) stimulus. Other models focus on the consequence of the action, whether pleasant or otherwise. This adds another component to learning – Stimulus>Response>Outcome. Examples of theories that look at learning in this way are 'instrumental conditioning' (Thorndike, 1913) and 'operant conditioning' (Skinner, 1953).

An environmental event (e.g. a patient having a cardiac arrest) may act as a stimulus, and the outcome of the individual's response to the stimulus can be either negative or positive. An example of a positive outcome to this environmental situation could be that the student found they were able to respond quickly to deliver basic life support even though they had not undertaken this in practice before. A possible negative outcome could be when a student responds by freezing and moving away from the patient, not instituting basic life support.

Reinforcement will lead to a change in behaviour, either to increase or decrease the likelihood of the behaviour recurring. In the previous example of a positive outcome from the student's response to a stimulus, the student is likely to develop increased confidence in their basic life support skills. Rewards such as feeling more confident in their practice or being praised by the mentor are examples of 'reinforcers' for a desired behaviour.

əɬɔ**Я****Reflective activity**

Being asked to carry out 'basic' care whilst an opportunity to develop clinical skills is missed could be regarded as a negative outcome and lead to a range of behaviours. Think about what behaviours the student might increase or decrease as a result of this negative situation, and what further actions this could lead to.

Behaviourist learning focuses on observable behaviours that occur as a result of consequences or beliefs and achieving goals or objectives, so you can see why many educators view learning in this way. The development of pre-specified objectives for educational experiences is based on behaviourist theories of learning and these are the basis for reliable and valid educational planning and assessment. The central contention is that educational goals should be specified beforehand and the way to assess learning should also be expressed in terms of observable and measurable behaviour. The arguments for pre-specifying objectives to direct and measure learning are powerful; however, there are objections. A behaviourist view of human beings, learning and the nature of knowledge can be seen as manipulative and as taking focus away from the personal, active, individual aspects of learning which can be intrinsically valuable.

Table 2.1 includes the names of some theorists who have investigated this approach to learning. Behaviourism has been much criticised, even after recent revisions, for falling short in its understanding of human personalities and different responses. It is difficult for this approach to learning to explain why some people continue to display negative behavioural responses.

əɬɔ**Я****Reflective activity**

Do you identify individual, personal objectives for learning in practice, or do you concentrate only on learning objectives defined by the educational programme for placement learning?

Educational programmes based on behaviourist views of learning might be competence based and promote standardisation of practice.

Key points Top tips

- Activity is important
- Frequent practice and repetition help in generalising and discriminating
- Reinforcement is the main motivating force
- Learning is helped by clear objectives

Table 2.1 Learning theories, theorists and the role of the mentor/clinical supervisor

Theory	Behaviourist	Cognitive	Humanistic
Theorists	Skinner Thorndike Watson	Bruner Gagné Piaget	Knowles Maslow Rogers
Role of the mentor	Learning outcome setter Behaviour modifier	Role model Disseminator of information Prompter	Facilitator Coach Listener

Cognitive theory

Cognitive theorists view learning as coming from experience, reasoning and the remembering of information that allows a person to adapt to the environment. Learning is about knowing, discovering and making meaning through intellectual processing and mental structuring. Understanding learning requires the study of information processing, as learning requires varying levels of elaboration moving from perception to the making of meaning. Remembering can be enhanced when, through experience, a person adds more connections to a single concept.

The cognitive processes that are the basis of the differing developmental stages between infancy and adulthood and from novice to expert have been studied. There has been significant interest in how some people learn new subjects and solve new problems more expertly than most, regardless of how much previous knowledge they have, i.e., intelligent novices. Understanding the way that these people control and monitor their thought processes will, it is hoped, identify ways of encouraging **metacognition,** an important lifelong learning skill. (Further exploration of learning from novice to expert is included in Chapter 8.)

Cognitive theories of learning are linked to 'Constructivism' which maintains that by reflecting on our own understanding of the world we

○━ℸ *Keywords*

Metacognition
The ability to think about thinking, to be consciously aware of ourselves as problem solvers, and to monitor and control our mental processing

develop our own rules, mental models and meanings. Learners are not seen as simply absorbing information but making tentative interpretations of experiences that they then elaborate on within their context. Feedback on learning is, therefore, internal to the individual. Cognitive theorists, with their concern for thinking processes, perception and intellectual functioning, have a less restrictive view of learning objectives. Objectives are seen as developmental as well as outcome based, representing learning journeys and negotiated between the learner and the mentor or clinical supervisor.

For example, when a student undertakes a new wound dressing they may bring to mind relevant prior learning and experiences, concerning infection control and wound care, and seek support from their mentor. They might refer to a clinical policy or procedure that has a structured presentational format. Opportunities to repeat this wound-care management will allow the student to strengthen their learning.

Educational programmes based on cognitive learning theories will be organised to provide opportunities to repeat and build on learning, and teach problem-solving approaches. Such programmes enable the learner to develop critical (commonly convergent) thinking, including the cognitive processes for making and evaluating decisions, and creative (commonly divergent) thinking, allowing the generation of ideas and innovative alternatives.

Key points   *Top tips*

- Teaching should be logical, structured and well organised
- Learner perceptions and prior knowledge are important
- Individual differences and approaches to thinking have a bearing on learning
- Learning *with* understanding is necessary

⚷ Keywords

Phenomenogical

Phenomenology takes the intuitive experience of phenomena (what presents itself to us in conscious experience) as its starting point and tries to extract from it the essential features of experiences and the holistic essence of what we experience

Self-actualisation

An individual is able to fully use and express their talents, capabilities and potential

Humanistic view of learning

From this perspective, the focus is on personal growth, the development of self-direction and interpersonal relationships. Behaviours are viewed as intentional and based on values, so to understand learning we need to study a person holistically as they grow and develop throughout their life. Feedback about learning is internal to the 'self' and based on individual motivations, goal setting and areas of interest. As learning is understood to be subjective, individual and based on experience, this way of looking at learning can alternatively be called **phenomenogical**. Learning has as its ultimate goal **self-actualisation**, not just behavioural change but changes in values, attitudes and beliefs.

Humanism is often linked to the adult education movement and the concept of andragogy. Andragogy has been defined as the 'art and science' of helping adults to learn. The term 'lifelong learning' rejects the model of education that is confined to childhood and early adulthood. Andragogy is based on six main assumptions (Knowles, 1990):

1   Adults need to know *why* they need to learn something.
2   Adults have a self-concept where they are responsible for their decisions and need to be treated in a way that acknowledges this self-direction.
3   Adult learners bring a wealth of previous experience to their current learning.
4   Adults are ready to learn something that has relevance to their everyday life.
5   Adults tend to be 'problem centred' in their learning.
6   Motivation mainly comes from 'internal' pressures, e.g. increased job satisfaction, self-esteem, and quality of life.

Knowles (1990) views an adult learner as having the following characteristics. They:

- respond best to a non-threatening learning environment where there is a good teacher–learner relationship
- want to assess themselves against a relevant standard to determine educational needs
- want to select their own learning experiences – self-directing
- prefer a problem-orientated, patient-based approach to learning
- want to apply their knowledge and skills immediately
- want to know how they are progressing
- want to contribute from their own knowledge and skills to help others to learn.

Although this view of adult learners still has some relevance (Knowles, 1990), the view has been much criticised, particularly for the implied absence of self-directed and problem-based learning from the area of children's learning (Tennant, 2005). There is still, I feel, a need to view adults as actively engaged in continuing education over time and in a range of settings and to see learning through continuous education as integral to all the roles that people undertake throughout their life. Education and learning is about dialogue, about giving the student the space and support to develop their ideas and themselves, within their social, political and economic context.

Humanistic-based educational programmes are learner centred, encourage reflection on personal experience, give some freedom and choice as to content, call for collaborative learning and are delivered in a non-threatening, facilitative environment. These programmes are less likely to have detailed, pre-set objectives, and the goals may continually be in the process of modification. Maslow (1970) sees goal formation as a highly dynamic process occurring through the learner's unique interaction with their experience.

Key points Top tips

- Goals of learning need to be personally relevant to the learner
- Personal learning is more important than knowledge acquisition
- Self-awareness and self-evaluation are important to learning
- Learning is a context-based natural process

Comparing the three approaches

If we take a nursing handover from one shift to another as an example of clinical practice, we can illustrate how these different approaches to learning might be viewed (see Table 2.2).

Table 2.2 Learning to undertake 'handover' of a shift

Behaviourism	Cognitivism	Humanism
The learner is 'conditioned' to undertake handover in a certain way that the rest of the profession has adopted in the locality (recognises this, knows what to do, presents handover information as others do).	The learner is encouraged to develop a structure to their handover that can be adapted when they meet an unfamiliar situation (extrapolates and knows how to deal flexibly with the changed circumstance).	The learner comes across a situation where one of the patients whom they are discussing at handover appears distressed as the patient's care is discussed at the bedside (formulates and reflects on the patient's feelings and their actions and feelings in response).

These three learning theories tend to focus on the individual, and learning is seen as being dependent on experiences. (Further exploration of learning from experience is included in Chapter 7.)

Recently, there has been increased interest in learning as a social and situational process. Learning is enhanced through social participation. Observation and interaction within a social context, between people and the environment, is seen as the basis of learning. (Further exploration of situated learning and communities of practice is included in Chapter 4.)

Types of knowledge

The process of learning is affected by conceptions of knowledge. The following level descriptors (Baxter Magolda, 1992) have been offered as a way to pick out varying levels of learning.

1 **Absolutist**. Knowledge is certain: 'I have to see what I'm learning about someone doing a patient assessment, and to know why I'm learning this.'

2 **Transition stage**. Partial certainty and uncertainty: 'Being shown two methods of undertaking a patient assessment, which both appear successful, changes your views on the 'right way' to handle a patient assessment.'

3 **Independent knowing**. Learning is uncertain and everyone has their own beliefs: 'I take things in by watching others and hearing their opinions on how I might improve my patient assessment skills, but I decide what I want and what I don't want to do.'

4 **Contextual knowing.** Knowledge is constructed and any judgement is made on the basis of evidence within a context: 'As I listen to the discussion regarding patient assessment, and think about my own experiences and others' viewpoints, I start to decide what I really think is important in this particular context.'

Reflective activity

Look at the level descriptors and the examples added regarding patient assessment and think about your own learning history. Can you identify a time in your life when your learning was absolutist, transitional, etc.? Did your age and the context that you were in at the time affect this?

Health care professionals require different kinds of knowledge. Evidence-based practice is a form of codified or empirical knowledge, defined by peer-reviewed research and published in books and journals, the 'gold standard' coming from randomised controlled trials. In order to approach care in an 'evidence-based' way, a practitioner needs to review the evidence available, thinking carefully and clearly about what makes most sense in influencing their clinical decisions. Wherever possible, scientific research that is relevant and properly conducted should be used. Evidence-based practice also means integrating individual clinical expertise with the best available external evidence.

Eraut (2000a) identifies cultural knowledge, located in space and time and interpreted differently by different groups, and personal knowledge which individuals bring to practical situations to help them think and perform. Phillips *et al.* (2000a) suggest that nurses make decisions through 'situated understanding' within practice settings.

There can be tensions between evidence-based practice and pragmatic practice. A knower's capacity to think and act is enhanced by the learning involved in making a 'scientific' concept available for use in a situation (Eraut, 2000b). However, even where research is reliable it may not be used in practice settings. The ability to make changes in practice is based on knowledge of the evidence available, and on learning from past experience. This is a complex art. The range of forms of knowledge and how they mix together is of great importance. It is recognised that Carper's (1978) empirical category of knowledge (she termed this 'scientific way of knowing') is supplemented by knowledge arising from:

- the art of performing clinical skills (aesthetic)
- the way nurses view and use themselves through being open to and focusing on the patient (personal)
- understanding the other person through recognising one's own experiences (personal)
- handling practice dilemmas and making moral decisions through moment-to-moment judgements about what should be done, what is right, and what is responsible (ethical).

Observation of nurse–patient interactions reveals all of these in action. It is, therefore, unlikely that only one way of 'knowing' would be informing the way that a nurse acts.

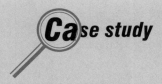
Case study

Forms of knowledge that inform professional working

Jane, a newly qualified staff nurse, is doing the post-operative observations for a woman who has returned after varicose veins surgery. A senior registered nurse is there watching her do the initial assessment. The newly qualified staff nurse is seeking approval for her work and for any omissions to be highlighted. She says, 'I'm not familiar with these forms.' The senior nurse shows her where to fill in the forms and sanctions her actions in disregarding certain parts of the form. She says, 'These are a bit more difficult. You could leave these as this is not applicable to day surgery – just make sure the wound is OK, and record the critical clinical data.'

What sorts of knowledge do you think are informing the junior and senior registered nurses' actions?

Aesthetics is the art of health care which involves seeing situations as a whole, not as component parts. It is the way that practitioners express and make their practice visible; through actions, bearing, conduct, attitudes, and interactions with patients. Carper (1978) suggests that aesthetics involves what is possible, not necessarily what is concrete, as the individual reflects on alternative courses of action. This way of knowing includes what is learnt as a result of professional experiences.

It is how a practitioner selects from their total knowledge and builds upon a wealth of experience in order to perform the 'art-act' (Jacobs-Kramer and Chinn, 1988). Often, this process of engaging, interpretation, and envisioning is unconscious or intuitive and mainly portrayed in narratives of critical incidents and reflections on care decisions.

An appreciation of the importance of all these forms of knowledge partly explains the cynicism from some practitioners regarding the potential impact of evidence-based practice. However, in many situations common sense and opinions are not a good enough basis for making decisions or developing understanding. For example, in deciding which drug to prescribe the practitioner would need knowledge from all the domains identified by Carper (1978). Poor professional practice would be displayed if he or she prescribed a drug regimen that there was strong evidence to suggest was not appropriate. In addition, there is a need for informed consent about the drug treatment and to have an awareness of the individual and their ability to comply with the medical treatment regimen.

When you think about the ways in which context affects your learning, you may have identified the role of emotion in learning; recently, there has been increasing interest in the relationship between feelings and learning. Goleman (1995) coined the term 'emotional intelligence' to encompass the understanding and learning about self and others' emotions that guides effective decisions. Managing personal emotions in an intelligent way requires self-awareness, impulse control, persistence, motivation, empathy and social deftness. The ability to manage personal emotions and the emotions of others is seen as an important facet of health care practice.

For instance, when a student health care practitioner has to deal for the first time with a dying or dead patient, there will be a range of factors influencing their learning about this new area of clinical practice. These include their:

● conception of the learning process/learning habits
● course teaching/assessment requirements
● perception of this area of clinical practice
● personal prior knowledge
● emotional response and how they manage self in relation to this aspect of practice
● experience of the current clinical environment
● conception of the structure of their knowledge.

These factors ultimately determine what the individual learns and the approach that they adopt to learning. They may focus on the superficial or surface characteristics of learning, for example, how to 'lay out' a body in line with the clinical guidelines, or on meaningful, deep learning, such as reflecting on their role within the health care team in maintaining a dying person's dignity and meeting their needs.

Evidence base

Read: Hopkinson, J. (2002) The hidden benefit: the supportive function of the nursing handover for qualified nurses caring for dying people in hospital. *Journal of Clinical Nursing*, **11** (2), 168–75.

Lifelong learning

Lifelong learning has been defined as a process of accomplishing personal, social and professional development (including formal, non-formal and informal learning) throughout the lifespan of the individual in order to enhance the quality of life of individuals and communities. Lifelong learning makes an assumption that learning takes place in all spheres of life, not just within educational institutes or in educational programmes. Lifelong learning is an important part of government policy related to a concern about the general skill and qualification levels of the economically active population. It is widely recognised that people will need continually to update and learn new skills if they are to remain competitive in the labour market. Titmus (1999) defines lifelong learning as the acquisition of learning skills for the immediate future, the ability to adapt such skills to meet the requirements of changing circumstance and applying learning to actions in a self-directed fashion.

Even though **self-directed learning** can be viewed as individual, self-directed adults use social networks and peer groups for emotional and educational support and guidance.

⚷ Keywords

Self-directed learning
The process by which adults take control of their own learning; in particular, how they set their own learning goals, locate resources, decide on which learning methods to use and evaluate their progress

Over to you

Look at the characteristics of the lifelong learner outlined in the following table (adapted from ENB, 1994). In your own experience, and based on past learning, can you think of examples from your practice that might illustrate that you are already a lifelong learner?

Try to identify an example for each of the characteristics.

Innovative in your practice	
Flexible to changing demands	
Resourceful in your methods of working	
Able to work as a change agent	
Able to share good practice and knowledge	
Adaptable to changing health care needs	
Challenging and creative in your practice	
Self reliant in your way of working	
Responsible and accountable for your work	

- What characteristics did you find more difficult to write about?
- Why do you think that was?
- What does this tell you about your personal philosophy of practice?
- What could you do with the information you have just generated?

Gopee (2002) looked at human and social capital as facilitators to lifelong learning. He suggests that 'human capital' (the investment by employers and employees in personal and professional development activities) is interrelated with 'social capital' (the time, patience and teaching that colleagues invest in each other within the social group). Therefore, learning is not just the accumulation of individual 'human capital', but is a benefit to a community through the sharing of knowledge gained from continuous professional activities, conferences, workshops, by peers and expert practitioners (Gopee, 2002).

It has been argued that there is a significant and positive correlation between professional development and autonomy and recognition, role clarity, job satisfaction, quality of supervision, peer support and opportunities for learning (Hart and Rotem, 1995). Practitioners practise in an environment of constant change and, to help ensure that lifelong learning is occurring, they are required to develop and keep a portfolio of learning (termed 'a personal professional profile') and are encouraged to access clinical supervision.

Continuous professional development

Before the 1990s, the majority of health care professionals' training focused on teaching routines and skills rather than on the ability to problem solve, rationalise the care given and exercise individual professional judgement. The increase in health care technology and the culture of constant change that is now synonymous with health care has influenced the need for increasingly competent and flexible professionals. Health care professionals have to provide some evidence of keeping themselves competent and up to date with their client care through continuous professional development (CPD).

CPD is:

> . . . a range of learning activities through which professionals maintain and develop throughout their career to ensure that they retain their capacity to practise safely, effectively and legally within their evolving scope of practice.
>
> (Health Professions Council, 2004, 1.2, p. 7)

CPD learning activities include:

- work-based learning, e.g. reflective practice, clinical audit, significant event analysis, user feedback, memberships of working groups/committees, journal club
- professional activity, e.g. member of a specialist interest group, mentoring, teaching, expert witness, presentations at conferences
- formal activity, e.g. courses, undertaking research, distance learning, planning and running a course
- self-directed learning, e.g. reading journals, articles, reviewing books, updating knowledge via the Internet, TV, press
- other activities, e.g. public service.

The way in which you take part in CPD will depend on your experiences and opportunities at work, profession or speciality, personal learning style, individual learning needs and the context of your practice.

Reflective activity

Take a blank sheet of paper and draw your professional time line starting when you first went into health care. Identify key learning events and changes to your professional working and experiences.

Nurses have been found to move frequently within the early years of their career, not in a 'migrant certificate gathering way', but getting good all round experience, actually creating pathways of professional development for themselves (Davies, 1995). Effective CPD has been linked with raised staff morale and increased motivation and is associated with staff retention (Mackereth, 1989). However, owing to methodological difficulties, there is a lack of conclusive evidence establishing a positive relationship between CPD and tangible improvements in patient care (Dowswell *et al.*, 1998; Wildman *et al.*, 1999), as many studies are based on the self-reports of learners (Smith and Topping, 2001).

Smith and Topping's (2001) case study of a group of post-registration paediatric learners showed that nurses had taken the course for many reasons, including to improve their knowledge, improve their patient care, enhance career opportunities, improve their interprofessional relationships, increase their confidence and to help them act as a knowledge resource for others. Nurses' choice of course was underpinned by a need for the course to be relevant to their work and of personal interest. Although CPD was generally valued, individuals within this case study talked about their frustration in trying to put into practice changes in clinical care in a context where there were staffing shortages (Smith and Topping, 2001).

Continuous professional development is seen as essential for sustaining and improving the quality of professional work, and much CPD is based within practice (Eraut, 1994). Technological competence is often a key aim in undertaking post-registration courses, and nurses advocated acquiring this in the clinical context (Little, 1999). A specialist clinical course led to increased self-confidence in the nurses' standards of care and a more questioning attitude to the practice of others (Wood, 1998). Students' 'perceived benefit' from the course could, however, be no more than a 'feel good' factor on completion of a course (Wigens and Westwood, 2000). Specialist post-registration courses, assessed in practice, allow qualified practitioners to focus time on their own learning needs, giving unspoken 'permission' to ask questions of both nursing and medical colleagues (Little, 1999, p. 70).

Despite changes in course delivery and assessment, including problem-based learning and portfolio assessment of practice, some nurses have been found to have negative views of CPD. Courses available at post-registration level are viewed by some as lacking a comprehensive and responsive approach to practitioners' needs (DoH, 1999; Robinson *et al.*, 2003). This was perhaps linked to a sense of CPD not being valued, in terms of the allocation of study time and financial support, and the perception that this affected career progression (Robinson *et al.*, 2003). It is argued that a flexible qualification system is required, with specialist qualifications that are updated when needed, and assessment systems that are capable of recording achievement beyond competence (Eraut, 1994). The concepts of lifelong learning and CPD integrate with ideas about organisational learning; encouraging learning within organisations is developed further in Chapter 10.

RRRRRRapid recap

Check your progress so far by working through each of the following questions.

1 What are the key differences between outcome-based and process-based learning?

2 List the key principles underpinning:
   (a) behaviourist theories of learning
   (b) cognitive theories of learning
   (c) humanistic theories of learning.

3 Explain the concepts 'lifelong learning' and 'continuous professional development'.

4 Why is it useful to be able to document learning through practice?

If you have difficulty with one of these questions, read through the section again to refresh your understanding before moving on.

3
Clinical placement areas

Learning outcomes

By the end of this chapter you should be able to:

★ Explain the code/guidelines for practice placements

★ Critically assess and evaluate a clinical area as a learning environment

★ Appreciate ways of getting the most from clinical environments, e.g. hub and spoke, teaching and learning programmes

★ Guide work-based learning.

Introduction

In this chapter we take a look at clinical placements, and clinical settings in general, to work out what issues impact on learning through practice. Health care professional students work in a variety of clinical settings, and individual experiences can affect perceptions of different specialities and different professions. The aim of the chapter is for you to appreciate the importance of formal and informal learning within clinical settings.

Health care professionals can bemoan the lack of time for teaching in clinical settings, and, when evaluating a clinical placement, students sometimes say that they have learnt little because there were no formal teaching sessions. These perceptions of learning fail to acknowledge that a stimulating clinical environment allows a great deal of informal learning to take place. Even so, effective learning in clinical practice does require the structured management of the following:

1 identifying learning needs
2 specifying learning objectives
3 determining available learning resources, experiences and strategies
4 agreeing evidence of accomplishment of learning objectives
5 specifying how the evidence will be validated
6 reviewing and assessing learning
7 evaluating the learning environment.

Structuring clinical learning

The first clinical placement has a powerful influence on confirming the health care career choice made by a student. Recognising the importance of a structured approach to practice learning can, therefore, be influential in retaining students.

> ## *Evidence base*
>
> Read: Chesser-Smyth, P. (2005) The lived experiences of general student nurses on their first clinical placement: A phenomenological study. *Nurse Education in Practice*, **5**, 320–7.

Through in-depth interviews with nursing students in Ireland, Chesser-Smyth (2005) found that:

> Although the initial observation stage (on a first placement) appears to last approximately two weeks, it was only when students became actively involved in the workload together with the acquisition of new knowledge that confidence levels increased and anxiety reduced.
>
> (Chesser-Smyth, 2005, p. 326)

O━┱ *Keywords*

Reality shock
The conflict caused by the movement from the familiar higher education environment to the unfamiliar work setting, caused by a gap between what has been learnt and on-the-job experiences

Many students may experience '**reality shock**' (Kramer, 1974) when they move out of the skills laboratories into clinical areas, and students may feel that they need to relearn skills. The stages of reality shock have been defined by Kramer (1974), in the following way:

1   Honeymoon – the student is fascinated with the new work.
2   Shock/Rejection – the student rejects the new environment, or the old environment, or self and may become socially isolated.
3   Recovery – the student is able to see the funny side of this, and is becoming competent.
4   Resolution – the student is able to display culturally appropriate reactions.

Added to this, students often compare their own practice with that of more experienced nurses, and this reinforces a lack confidence in their own abilities.

Professional confidence is thought to underpin clinical competency (Bell *et al.*, 1998) and a positive change in the confidence of nursing students has a significant impact on their performance within practice (Ferguson, 1996). Clinical educators identify role-modelling, discussion, commitment and mutual respect as key ways of promoting confidence, whereas students suggest that encouragement, goodwill, acting as a resource/role model and promoting patient care are important (Flagler *et al.*, 1988). Crooks *et al.* (2005) noted that students developed their professional confidence through becoming informed, finding a voice of their own to discuss their clinical practice, becoming self-directed in their learning and by comparing their care delivery with that of other colleagues at work. Confident mentors/supervisors who are comfortable with supporting, challenging and extending students' learning, and are available to supervise regularly, are the basis of good-quality practice teaching. The work area needs to appreciate the practice teaching component within a practitioner's workload and the time that undertaking this role requires.

Learning needs are identified by the gap between where the learner is presently and where they want to be. This may involve analysing the skills and knowledge required in performing a particular task or job and identifying where the person stands at the moment in relation to the level of knowledge and skills. Resources required to carry this out should be identified, and steps on the way to achieving the learning outcomes can be agreed. In some clinical settings, this takes the form of a learning contract. A learning contract is an individualised learning plan that should be negotiated between the mentor/supervisor and the learner. It specifies what the student will learn, the time span, how learning will be achieved, and the criteria for measuring success. Using a learning contract hands over the control of learning to the student and modifies the power relations between the assessor and the student. It is important that the learner and mentor/supervisor identify what the learner should be able to demonstrate to show achievement of the learning outcomes. What this evidence looks like then becomes the specific focus of the placement/clinical learning.

Opportunities need to be provided for students to observe safely, rehearse and demonstrate these skills. A variety of methods, including experiential and practice-based learning are employed by the mentor/supervisor to guide the student towards competence. Experiences in practice settings require effective facilitation to meet the desired learning outcomes. To try to help with the structuring of the learning opportunity during a clinical placement, it can be useful to think about the five main approaches to this:

- clinical work with a mentor/supervisor/other
- observing the practice of experienced practitioners
- researching an evidence base for practice in the placement
- a learning pack related to the clinical setting
- thinking of the placement area as a 'hub' and arranging 'spoke' experiences, e.g. visits to other departments, spending time with specialist clinicians (Channell, 2002).

Health care professions are practice-based disciplines and so learning occurs primarily in clinical settings with qualified practitioners acting as role models. Skills and values are projected and learnt, largely subconsciously, during practitioners' everyday work. Clinical teaching is, therefore, an integral part of the qualified professionals' role. Fundamental and specific skills to be developed to improve clinical teaching include the following:

Fundamental clinical teaching skills

- Relationship building
- Negotiating learning contracts
- Questioning
- Active listening
- Challenging
- Reflection skills
- Preparation for learning
- Support skills
- Catalytic skills
- Giving information and advice
- Giving feedback

Further discussion regarding these skills is presented in Chapter 6.

Health care professionals are often inherently good teachers and communicators. They spend a great deal of time teaching patients, family, support staff and other health care professionals. Teaching students in the clinical situation is an aspect of professional development; it requires refining of those teaching skills to cover a variety of scenarios. A short description of a clinical learning situation is included here for you to reflect on the 'key learning issues'. There are no 'correct' answers, but this activity should help you to examine your opinions and values regarding teaching and learning in the clinical environment.

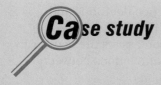

Case study

Welcoming and orientating a student to a new clinical area

The student arrives on the first day of the placement. She has not visited the area beforehand and only has the name of the mentor, whom she approaches. The mentor, standing with arms folded, says that she was not expecting any new student today, but that's not untypical for the way the higher education institute arranges allocations. The mentor suggests that the student settles in by watching how things are done as it is very busy today.

1 How would you have felt if you were this student?

2 Whose responsibility is it in your clinical area to plan a student's orientation?

3 What could the mentor have done to get the placement off to a better start? Identify the negative non-verbal behaviours.

4 In what ways do non-verbal behaviours from a mentor or clinical supervisor affect a student's behaviours and thinking processes?

Having thought about the initial welcome that a student receives from a mentor or supervisor on their first day in a new practice setting, you may have formed a concept of the key facets of a structured and competent orientation meeting.

Competence includes a broad range of knowledge, attitudes and observable patterns of behaviour which together form the ability to deliver a specified professional service. Many ways have been tried to undertake assessment of clinical skills including:

- simulation
- video testing
- objective structured clinical examination (OSCE)
- observation during 'real practice'.

Obviously, within the placement environment the key feature is the ability to observe and deliver 'real' practice. Students learn in the 'real situation', where the theory they have learnt becomes 'meaningful'. Indeed, when considering learning skills for practice, some theorists suggest that 'skills can only be learnt as an integrated whole in the clinical environment' (Eraut, 1994). This is one example of why the learning that takes place in practice is so important. Clinical areas are busy and, although mentors and supervisors work with students, there are occasions when students may work with unqualified staff or on their own because clinical areas are often short staffed. This makes learning clinical skills difficult at times.

One conceptual model suggested for promoting learning in clinical contexts is the 'Partner, Learn, Progress' model (Henderson *et al.*, 2006). Within this model, the terms indicate the following:

- Partner – the positive, trusting relationship developed between an experienced practitioner and the learner. Although this is at an interpersonal level, this will be affected by the broader social context, such as the clinical team.

- Learn – the experienced practitioner helps the learner to make sense of all the forms of knowledge that inform practice decisions and delivery: knowledge that may have seemed to the learner to be distant from practice. This mutual collaboration assists the learner in practising safely within the context, making connections between meanings, experiences, feelings and attitudes.

- Progress – the previous two components of the model allow the learner (and the experienced practitioner) to develop their knowledge further.

All students are allocated a named mentor/supervisor who should have appropriate experience of their working environments and meet the necessary requirements as set out by the appropriate professional governing bodies. Mentors/supervisors should guide students for a length of time that is sufficient to enable them to make an informed judgement about students' performance and achievement.

Whenever a mentor/supervisor meets a learner it is useful to structure the meeting appropriately. An example of a possible framework is given below.

Key points | **Top tips**

Framework for meeting with a learner:
1 Think about the introduction and purpose of the meeting
2 Take time to put the learner at ease
3 Explain how the meeting will be recorded
4 Ask generally about how it is going
5 Ask about their practice learning, work/study patterns and if they have any problems
6 Review their assessment work so far
7 Deal with any specific issues the learner wants to raise
8 Discuss the arrangements for follow-up/further meetings

Normally the student and mentor/supervisor should have at least three formal meetings during a clinical placement; guidance for the content of these is given below.

Content of formal meetings

Initial meeting
- To identify the student's learning needs.
- To discuss the learning opportunities available to the student.
- To identify the knowledge and skills available for practice development and assessment.

The student and mentor/supervisor should leave the meeting with enough information to develop their plans, which will be reviewed at the interim/midpoint meeting.

Midpoint meeting
- To review the student's progress in relation to the learning outcomes/plan.
- To identify areas where the student is progressing well and is expected to achieve.
- To identify areas where the student is not progressing as expected and to develop a further action plan to support the student's additional learning needs.

The mentor/supervisor should determine whether additional support should be sought e.g. clinical placement facilitator, link lecturer.

Final assessment meeting
- To assess the student's overall performance, in relation to the learning outcomes and grading criteria.
- To evaluate the clinical placement learning.

The meeting should be handled in such a way that there is closure. Even though this may not be done on the final placement attendance this should be planned for the final week.

A 'critical mass' of placements and assessors appears to be an important factor in sustaining health care programmes over time. Those employers who are able to offer large numbers of placements on a regular basis often have large numbers of assessors and experienced staff. If a placement has few assessors, the student may be assessed using a 'long-arm' approach where an off-site assessor oversees the assessment by working with the staff who supervise directly, on site.

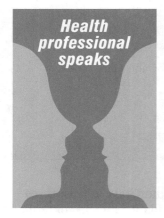

Health professional speaks

Link lecturer

We work on the principle that those who can practise can also clinically teach. Associate mentors/supervisors help with student support, assisting the qualified mentors/supervisors so there is almost a team approach to student support. These associate mentors offer support ranging from individual supervision, through joint assessment of the student, to 'arm's length' support as a member of the team. This model allows us to offer 'apprenticeships' to inexperienced assessors who want to develop their skills, as well as allowing other members of the multidisciplinary team to have involvement in the supervision of students from other health care professions. In this way we successfully create a large pool of mentors/assessors.

Lecturers may visit the clinical placement areas, although this varies depending on the health care programme. When a visit does occur, the purpose is mainly to establish that the students feel comfortable in the work setting and have access to the appropriate clinical experiences, and this should be established in a private conversation with the students. The visit also gives the opportunity for the placement staff to let the lecturer know whether they are happy with the placement arrangements, to discuss student performance and to identify any difficulties or issues that have arisen.

Key points **Top tips**

Top tips for mentors/supervisors:

- Assess your feelings about working with students
- Find out about the students with whom you are working
- Learn to combine giving care and teaching students at the same time
- When it is quiet, offer alternative learning experiences
- Communicate effectively and involve other colleagues, lecturers and practice educators
- Share the important characteristics of your practice, and how you make your clinical decisions with students

Learner responsibilities on placement

Overall, learning environments are viewed positively if students are encouraged to take responsibility for their own learning outcomes and are given protected learning time to achieve these. A student has responsibility to be proactive about their learning. Clinical staff can assist by answering questions but they will find it difficult and unrewarding to continue to give information if you show little interest. As a student, you can prepare yourself by reading appropriate texts about the clinical speciality and thinking about your needs in relation to the placement and to your stage of training. This will help you to reflect on the experience at a later date. Staff in clinical areas deal with many students and cannot be expected to remember all of an individual student's needs at a particular point in the student's training, especially in areas where there is a very fast throughput of patients. So students need to remind staff if they require a particular experience to achieve their learning outcomes.

An action plan is simply a list of things to be achieved, identifying how this will be done. Although it is common for supervisors to set objectives for learners, learners can also set objectives for themselves. It can help when writing these to begin by stating, 'After this experience/ placement I will be able to . . .' and then specify what will have been learnt. A set of objectives can also provide a valuable aid to reflection and self-assessment after the placement.

In addition, students need to perceive that their learning experiences are equitable in comparison with those of other students, and that they have received the appropriate mix of support and supervision from experienced and knowledgeable members of the multidisciplinary team.

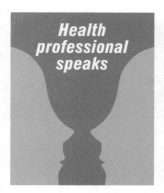

Health professional speaks

Student

The supervisor on my last placement was really helpful in making sure that I had the experiences I needed as a student, asking me specifically if there was something I wanted to do that I hadn't done yet. She made sure that if the opportunity arose I wouldn't miss out, by telling all the other staff. I really appreciated this compared to other placements where I received such a negative experience from people whom I asked for help.

Reflective activity

Compare two areas where you have had very differing levels of clinical practice facilitation and identify what you did differently in those practice areas.

Experience is gained through seeing how others do things, or what happens in a particular context; however, if you are new to a situation, you may not know what to look for, and it can be very easy to miss opportunities and to notice very little. This problem can be reduced by the use of a simple observation checklist that covers what to look out for and perhaps asks the learner to record events and how often they happened. Simple checklists can be devised by the learner or with the assistance of the mentor/supervisor. For example, prior to seeing a physiotherapist mobilising a patient for the first time following hip replacement surgery, the physiotherapist and the student or students could have a short discussion about what to look out for, and devise a brief checklist. Afterwards, the list could be used to structure a short discussion which encourages reflection on what has been seen and the significance that these observations have for future practice.

It can be difficult to undertake a task effectively if you do not have a sound understanding of what would count as doing it well. It makes an enormous difference to how attentive a learner is when undertaking a practical task if they have a clear idea of the criteria that will be used to judge the outcome of their work.

Many higher education institutes have developed their own student's charter which gives guidance about the learner's rights and responsibilities in relation to clinical practice. These are often written with involvement from placement providers as well as the health care teaching staff. If a student charter is available, both the mentor and student should be aware of its content.

Over to you

Find out if your locality has a student charter, and take a look at its content. Ask yourself if all of these standards are being met.

A health care student becomes closely involved with the public in a professional capacity and, therefore, should at all times work in a manner acceptable to the profession to which they aspire and follow the code of conduct. When on placement, the learner has access to confidential and personal information relating to patients/clients and sensitive information relating to other members of staff who are work colleagues. It is important to remember to maintain confidentiality even outside the clinical environment.

Reflective activity

Whilst travelling home on the bus from an early shift, you hear a member of staff discussing a patient whom they are treating. Although you do not know this health carer, you can identify the area/placement in which they work and the patient details being discussed are fairly specific. Think about what you could/might do.

- Have you ever experienced a situation where a student or colleague was not professional in their conduct, and how did this make you feel?
- How did you deal with the situation?

Whatever the dress code for the clinical area, the learner has a responsibility to adhere to this, promoting a professional image and keeping to health and safety policies. An identification badge should be worn at all times in clinical areas.

Different placement areas may vary in their working patterns and shifts, and the student should be made aware of these details prior to commencing the placement. The student will be expected to adopt the placement's duty rotas, which may include working early and late shifts, weekends, and night duty where this is the normal pattern of working. In many placements, the student is supernumerary and, therefore, takes on the same duty rota as their mentor or supervisor; however, adjustment may be made to ensure that the student has experience in all aspects of care within the speciality or to take account of the student's personal commitments. If a student is not working with their mentor/supervisor because of sickness or a differing shift pattern, the registered practitioner, who is responsible for that particular shift, acts as the associate mentor/supervisor.

All attendance on a placement should be recorded accurately to fulfil the requirements of the health care programme; there may be a specified number of clinical hours to be achieved by the end of a professional course. If the student is unable to attend a clinical placement as scheduled, they must inform the clinical staff prior to the start of the shift. Usually, in addition, the higher education institute also needs to be informed of any sickness or absence. The student should also inform the placement area and the higher education institute of their return from sickness or absence.

Students should keep themselves informed regarding placement allocations and any changes and should prepare for the impending speciality.

Clinical staff can provide mentorship, supervise the student's experience and assess their practice according to the requirements of their course. Health professionals, other than nurses and midwives and other members of staff all contribute to your learning experiences, so make sure that you engage with the multidisciplinary team.

The clinical learning environment

All learners and staff within clinical areas are adults. Having a concept of the adult learner (defined as andragogy and discussed in Chapter 2) may help in thinking about a particular clinical learning environment. Students' level of satisfaction is raised when they are treated with respect and as individuals (Randle, 2003). Students' needs should be considered within a well-managed and motivated clinical learning situation.

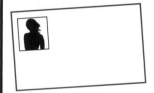

Clinical Caseload . . .

Answer the following questions about your current clinical area to determine the clinical teaching caseload and to assess the area as a clinical learning environment; where appropriate, identify action points.

1 Give a brief description of the practical experience offered in this area.

2 Is practice supported by high standards of documentation regarding client/patient care/treatment?

3 Are clinical governance arrangements in place to support evidence-based practice?

4 Is the environment physically, socially and psychologically safe for staff and clients/patients?

5 Are all mentors/supervisors familiar with the assessment strategy of students' courses?

6 Do mentors/supervisors get the opportunity to meet and work regularly with their students?

7 Are there sufficient mentors/supervisors to ensure appropriate levels of supervision? (Has the maximum number of students the area can supervise been identified, and the number of staff who are fully prepared for a supervision role?)

8 Are there effective communication channels between staff and clients?

9 Are policies/guidelines/protocols accessible and up to date?

10 Do students receive a 'welcome pack'/orientation on arrival in the area?

11 Do you receive formal and informal evaluations of the learning environment from students?

12 Does the practice experience enable students to gain experience of the role of qualified staff in a range of contexts?

13 Do students gain experience of working interprofessionally?

14 Is the clinical team spirit motivated towards developing students' learning?

15 What learning/facilitation roles are available for students, e.g. mentor/preceptor/clinical supervisor; practice educator; teacher/lecturer/tutor; others?

Question 14 asked you to assess the clinical team spirit: team spirit does impact on the overall learning environment (Wigens, 2004); however, it is important to remember that a popular placement is not necessarily synonymous with an effective learning environment although there are obvious advantages.

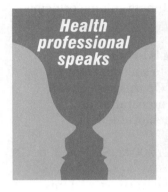

Health professional speaks

Registered nurse

Being a student placement for third year students helps recruitment, both in a sense of bringing would-be employees into close contact with the team and so encouraging them to apply for vacancies, and also because it provides a hands-on opportunity for us to experience the work of the would-be applicants.

Having started to identify the strengths and weaknesses in the clinical area in which you are presently working, it is perhaps useful to see what researchers have found out about the vital elements for good placement learning experiences. Papp *et al.* (2003) and Koh (2002), researching in Finland and England respectively, found that there needed to be high levels of co-operation between staff members, enhanced care standards, and a good atmosphere where students are regarded as colleagues. Students wanted to feel appreciated for their contribution to clinical practice and to feel part of the team, and their supervisor/mentor is vital in assisting with this. The clinical setting is often changing and sometimes unpredictable, which can make it hard to plan an optimal clinical learning environment for students. Even so, from your previous review of the learning environment, you can probably identify some areas for improvement.

Over to you

Improvement action plan: having thought about your current workplace/placement as a learning environment, what would be the first thing you would do to bring about improvements? Draw up a list of achievable steps aimed at prioritising and implementing your improvements.

It is essential that arrangements are made to ensure that issues of ethnicity, disability and gender are taken account of during the placement, so that there is evidence that the requirements of equal opportunities/equalities policies are met on an ongoing basis.

Mechanisms to ensure placements are effective

Clinical placements are considered to be the most influential aspects of nurse education programmes, and this is likely to be the case for many health care programmes. To allow student nurses to meet the National Midwifery Council (NMC) proficiencies and ensure that they are 'fit to practice', the NMC (2004a) states within its guiding principle for practice-centred learning that:

> The primary aim in pre-registration nursing is to ensure that students are prepared safely and effectively to such an extent that the protection of the public is assured. On this basis, it is a fundamental principle that programmes of preparation are practice-centred and directed towards the achievement of professional proficiency.
>
> (NMC, 2004a, Section 3, p. 13)

The clinical environment should ensure effective learning, and this includes strategies for quality assurance of standards, and the development of a change culture (NMC, 2002). Care in clinical placements needs to be evidence based and reflect respect for the rights of service users, including maintaining their dignity, privacy and religious needs. Students are exposed to a variety of care approaches, as each placement will have its own philosophy and model of care in use. However, every placement should adhere to all relevant local and governmental policies and procedures.

Placements must be effectively prepared for student allocation and should provide an equitable opportunity for each individual to achieve their respective placement outcomes. Institutions should ensure that students are provided with appropriate guidance and support in preparation for, during and after their placements; this includes:

- appropriate induction to the placement environment including health and safety information
- any occupational health, legal or ethical considerations or requirements (e.g. patient confidentiality)
- the means of recording the achievement of learning outcomes
- availability of additional skills preparation
- cultural orientation and work expectations
- institutional support services that students can access (QAAHE, 2001).

Students should be given an opportunity to evaluate a placement so that the clinical staff, managers and the higher education institute can work on the areas for improvement or celebrate and disseminate 'good practice'. This usually takes the form of a questionnaire, but is also strengthened by a discussion at the end of the placement period. The questionnaire usually focuses on the welcome received, the range of clinical experience gained, opportunities provided to communicate with staff and patients, whether the placement allowed achievement of the learning outcomes, the level of feedback and support from mentors/supervisors, and the availability and access to resources. These resources can be in the form of journals, other publications, the Internet, multidisciplinary forums, specialist 'spoke' placements and the physical space for the student and mentor to meet. The benefit of using a questionnaire, in addition to verbal feedback, is aided if the questionnaire is completed anonymously. Some higher education institutes add some free-text boxes for detailed comments on strengths and areas for improvement.

Many schools of nursing report that getting busy clinical staff and students to complete an evaluation tool is a perennial problem (Moseley *et al.*, 2004), so having an effective and simple tool is essential. Attempts

Table 3.1 Example of an evaluation of clinical placement questionnaire

1	During my first day/shift I was provided with a planned introduction to the practice placement area.
2	During my first day/shift I was allocated a supervisor/supervisory team.
3	A range of resources was available for my use in the placement area.
4	During my placement, the staff encouraged me to ask questions about practice/theory.
5	During my placement, staff used placement learning/teaching opportunities which supported my learning needs.
6	During my placement, staff encouraged and supported me to learn as and when the opportunities arose.
7	During my first day/shift, I was given the name of my mentor/supervisor.
8	In the first part of my placement, my mentor/supervisor and I discussed how I could achieve the required skills and learning outcomes for the placement.
9	My mentor/supervisor and I set target dates and reviewed my progress as required by my course and as appropriate to my length of placement.
10	During the placement, I received feedback on my progress and discussed this with my mentor/supervisor.
11	On completion of my placement, all relevant documentation was completed, signed and dated by my mentor/supervisor as required by my course (e.g. learning contract, skills book, portfolio).
12	During each shift I was supervised by either a named mentor/supervisor or a small supervisory team.
13	I was able to discuss my level of supervision with my mentor/supervisor.
14	At all times during the placement I knew who was supervising me.
15	Placement details were made available to me at least two weeks before the placement start date.

to improve the placement evaluation have been made (RCN, 2002a), and Moseley *et al.* (2004) have empirically tested their 15-statement tool in the UK, Finland and Germany. A numerical rating can be placed alongside these statements allowing the generation of computerised reports, and individual and cohort tracking.

Over to you

Take a look at the 15 statements included in the final tool (Moseley *et al.*, 2004). Note that I have adapted some of the wording (identified in italics).

- I got on well with the clinical staff.
- I had a good working relationship with the *mentor*/preceptor.
- Questions were answered satisfactorily.
- Staff explained procedures to me.
- I was treated as part of the team.
- The *mentor*/preceptor had a good sense of humour.
- Staff encouraged me to ask questions.
- The *mentor*/preceptor pointed out learning opportunities.
- Nurses gave me information about the care *that* they were giving to patients.
- The *mentor*/preceptor encouraged students to ask questions.
- The *mentor*/preceptor attached great importance to my learning needs.
- The more I put into the placement, the more I got out.
- I was motivated and keen to learn.
- Patients were well cared for.
- The *mentor*/preceptor was confident in *their* ability to teach me.

Compare the type of evaluative data that you would submit about your current placement/work area using this tool with the data that would be elicited by the questionnaire example given previously.

As well as the evaluation of the placement, there should also be a structured debriefing session after the placement so that students within a cohort gain maximum benefit from their placement experiences. Debriefing activities can take many forms including group discussion, patient/user involvement, presentations, and drama workshops. The key facet of this debriefing is that students can discuss and share their experiences, clarify and present their learning and identify areas for further knowledge development. Wherever possible, practice-based learning should dovetail with classroom-based learning.

RRRRR**Rapid recap**

Check your progress so far by working through each of the following questions.

1 Define the term 'reality shock' and identify the possible stages of this.

2 What should be the minimum number of formal meetings that a mentor/supervisor undertakes with a student, and what structure could be used for these meetings?

3 How should a student handle a period of sickness or absence from a placement area?

4 What guidance does the QAAHE think should be made available to all students attending a placement area?

If you have difficulty with one of these questions, read through the section again to refresh your understanding before moving on.

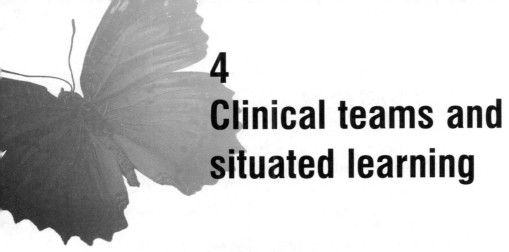

4
Clinical teams and situated learning

Introduction

In this chapter you will be thinking about the clinical teams and about situated learning in clinical environments. You will explore the relationship between participating in clinical practice and the social environment and learning.

Situated learning

Reflective activity

Have you ever sat in a classroom listening to a lecture and thought to yourself, 'What relevance has this to the real world of practice?' Think about one of these times and try to identify why you were thinking this and whether, with the benefit of hindsight, your opinion has changed.

A possible reason why you were uninspired by that lecture is that the content was not easily remembered and seemed unrelated to your future working. Some theories of learning are based on what has been described as a 'content fetish' (Gee, 2004). From this stance, physiotherapy or nursing, for example, is composed of a set of facts and skills – a body of knowledge – and learning occurs when this information is taught to an individual and then tested. Conventional theories view learning as a process of individual internalisation of knowledge; however, learning is also influenced by other people.

In the first chapter, you were introduced to the term situated learning and to situated understanding as a norm of everyday life. The question 'How are you today?' can mean different things in different contexts as people construct their own meaning from the social clues around them. The meaning of the communication and the expectations that it generates can be very different when 'How are you today?' is said in a ward setting, when someone appears distressed, compared with when it is used while passing an acquaintance in a hospital corridor. For some learning theorists (Lave and Wenger, 1991; Rogoff, 1990), any domain of knowledge is first and foremost a set of activities and experiences. For instance, nurses see, talk and do nursing when they are nursing and think about their interactions whilst nursing in a different way from non-nurses.

In developing the concept of the 'zone of proximal development' (ZPD), Vygotsky focused on the learning context as an important variable, shifting the emphasis from what has been learnt to learning capability (Cole *et al.*, 1978). Vygotsky suggested that a novice's development occurs through participation in activities beyond their competence with the assistance of skilled professionals who provide the 'scaffolding' for learning, and experts withdraw or 'fade' as increasing competency is shown by the novice (Rogoff, 1990).

There is a distinction between scientific knowledge and everyday concepts, and it is argued that maturity of learning is achieved when the scientific and everyday merge (Vygotsky, in Cole *et al.*, 1978). Engestrom (1994) expanded learning to include social transformation, covering all everyday actions from a wider historical and societal perspective. A key difference between Vygotsky's (in Cole *et* al., 1978) and Lave and Wenger's (1991) views on social learning relates to the internalisation of learning. Instead of viewing learning as internalisation, Lave and Wenger take a more radical perspective, seeing learning as the result of increasing participation in communities of practice. (Refer back to Chapter 1 for a definition of communities of practice.) The development of situated learning was a response to trying to understand early forms of **apprenticeship** where students spent their time, often a number of years, gradually acquiring knowledge and skills from an expert.

This form of learning was criticised as being context embedded, limited in scope, not sufficiently explicit, lacking in creativity, potentially out of date and as learning by rote. In a similar vein, clinical-based learning was traditionally a significant component of training for nursing and other health care professions but had been viewed as inferior to classroom-based higher education programmes. There is now increased acceptance of the situated nature of learning, and Lave and Wenger (1991) even go as far as to suggest that practical knowledge cannot be generalised or decontextualised.

Mikkelsen Kyrkjebø and Hage (2005) recognise that nursing students learn clinical practice from a range of communities of practice of very mixed quality. This can lead to the development of varying types of relationships between student health care practitioners and their clients; these relationships have been characterised as mechanistic, authoritative and facilitative (Suikkala and Leino-Kilpi, 2005).

- **Mechanistic relationship.** Students focus on their own needs, intent on acquiring knowledge and technical skills. External factors

⚷ *Keywords*

Apprenticeship
A period of time working for a skilled person, often for low payment, in order to learn that person's skills

such as the supervisor's daily routines and advice for performing physical tasks and aspects of care and treatment drive this type of relationship.

- **Authoritative relationship**. Students assume what is best for the patient and problem solve care; in some instances, patients are able to make decisions about their own care and treatment. Informal communications between the student and patient tend to be superficial.

- **Facilitative relationship**. Patient's expectations and requirements for care and treatment govern student interactions. Students and patients know each other personally and the relationship could be described as close and warm (Suikkala and Leino-Kilpi, 2005).

The student's ability to develop a facilitative relationship with patients is affected by many factors, both individual and within the **clinical milieu**. The caring attributes of student nurses develop throughout their three years of training and through the varying cultures within their placements (Suikkala and Leino-Kilpi, 2005).

It has been suggested that various factors can promote or impede good student–patient relationships. These are identified within Table 4.1.

O—π *Keywords*

Clinical milieu
The physical and social aspects of the clinical environment: in fact, the totality of the surroundings

Table 4.1 Factors promoting or impeding good student–patient relationships (adapted from Suikkala and Leino-Kilpi, 2005, p. 350)

Promoting factors	Impeding factors
Individual characteristics • positive way of thinking, expectations and attitude • intellectual and interpersonal competence	Individual characteristics • tendency to negativity or stereotyped expectations and attitudes • lack of intellectual and interpersonal competence
Patient-related factors • positive frame of mind • favourable demographic and diagnostic characteristics	Patient-related factors • tendency to negativity • unfavourable demographic and diagnostic characteristics
Length of time together • patients' long hospital stays • students' long clinical placements • workload allocation is patient centred	Length of time together • patients' short hospital stays • students' short clinical placements • workload high and task centred
Atmosphere • role models of staff relationships with patients are good • supportive supervisory relationship • positive and encouraging feedback from clinical team	Atmosphere • role models of staff relationships with patients are bad, lack of privacy during patient care and treatment • lack of supportive supervisory relationship • negative feedback from clinical team

In the following account, a health professional identifies how she came to limit and define her nurse–patient relationship by learning through practice.

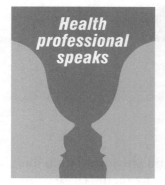

Health professional speaks

Registered nurse

During my training I was aware that I would occasionally get very attached to someone, particularly if I had done a lot of their care. I don't think you can opt to become involved although . . . During my training, we were told not to become too involved because we could become too stressed. I think that in the old-style training people were very worried that we'd get far too attached. I think I'm at a stage where I became involved to a point. Since I qualified I have become more experienced at dealing with it.

⊶ Keywords

Hidden curriculum
The unacknowledged, covert socialising processes of education that leads to the learning of cultural norms, values and beliefs

When you read what this nurse has to say about how she learnt about developing a nurse–patient relationship and about the comments from tutors and other health care staff to avoid 'getting too involved', what do you infer about the '**hidden curriculum**' at that time? This type of 'general rule' appeared to be of little use to her when she first went into clinical placements.

Marinker (1974) suggests that the hidden curriculum is learnt by observation and copying those around us. He stressed the importance of role models and the significance of mentors and supervisors reinforcing classroom messages through their clinical practice. The characteristics and behaviours of role models that were highly regarded by students include:

- effective practitioner
- learner- and patient-centred
- teamwork skills
- problem solver
- enthusiastic
- effective communicator
- leadership.

Obviously, the 'hidden curriculum' concept can also apply within patient teaching scenarios.

What follows is an excerpt from a two-hour antenatal class attended by a health visitor and a student nurse who was studying aspects of family health care; it was the third of six planned sessions with expectant mothers. The health visitor who had taught the first two sessions intended in this session to cover the role of the health visitor. The speaker's non-verbal behaviour is described within brackets.

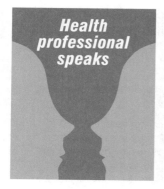

Health professional speaks

Health visitor

We're there to advise: never to tell you what to do. The health visitor takes over from the midwife and will do some home visits (sitting on the edge of the chair, feet crossed, leaning forward, holding teaching notes). We also have a baby clinic you can visit any time on Tuesday afternoon. Often people want information on weaning. What about breast-feeding? (looks around). You're all breast-feeding? We have good rates of breast-feeding in this area – although people sometimes struggle in the first couple of weeks. If you are unable to breast feed, baby milk is the next best thing.

The emotional incentives, hidden curriculum and pressures within the social setting may be visible. Having read the above excerpt, try to grasp the meaning, rules and roles being reinforced.

- Meanings are humanly constructed sets of concepts consciously singled out as important aspects of reality.
- Rules are shared meanings in a specific situation and their consequences.
- Roles are labels people use to organise activity and make sense of what applies to others and the consequences of this.

Key points | *Top tips*

- Situated learning contrasts with traditional classroom learning that involves knowledge presented in an abstract form or out of context
- Situated learning is a function of the activity, context and culture within which it occurs
- Learning can be incidental and requires social interaction and collaboration
- Knowledge needs to be presented in an authentic context

⚬⟵ Keywords

Professional socialisation

Professional socialisation is the process whereby newcomers to a profession acquire the values, attitudes, skills and knowledge that allow them to become a member of a professional subculture

It is useful in understanding situated learning to look briefly at the concept of **professional socialisation.**

Socialisation theories focus on how the individual achieves membership of a group by internalising its norms. Weidman *et al.* (2001) define professional socialisation as the process by which people acquire the knowledge, skills, and disposition that makes them more effective members of a group, and higher education is a first step in this process. Through the process of acquiring prescribed knowledge, the student also learns about appropriate professional behaviour and attitudes. Individuals are developing professional values that guide their behaviours and define their sense of belonging to a professional group. The prescribed knowledge consists of the theoretical body of knowledge, methods and technology, and the interaction of all these elements produces professional language.

The socialisation model presented by Weidman *et al.* (2001) has four components comprising professional socialisation:

1 prospective students (background, predisposition)
2 professional communities (practitioners, associations)
3 personal communities (family, friends and employers)
4 novice professional practitioners.

According to this model, the ultimate outcome is the professional who has transformed their self-image, attitudes and thinking processes. Upon qualification, professionals embark on two more socialisation processes: one into the organisation that employs them and the second into their profession.

Over to you

Read: MacKinnon, G., McAllister, D. and Anderson, S. (2001) Introductory practice experience: an opportunity for early professionalisation. *American Journal of Pharmaceutical Education*, **65**, 247–253.

MacKinnon *et al.* (2001) reported on the development, implementation and associated outcomes of a 30-week introductory practice course at Midwestern University College of Pharmacy, Glendale, in the United States. Do you concur with their findings that the introductory practice experiences were valuable in the early professionalisation of students?

Although professional socialisation is an aspect of situated learning, Wenger (1998) suggests that education needs to be understood as changing identity in a lifelong process, not merely in terms of an initial period of socialisation into a subculture, such as a profession. Learning through practice becomes a mutual development process between individuals and communities. There is a subtle difference between the imitation and internalisation of norms and the construction of identities within communities of practice.

Communities of practice

At any given time, you belong to a range of communities of practice – at home, at work and in relation to your hobbies. These communities of practice are integral to your daily living: an example might be the members of a scout group where you act as the scout leader every Friday.

The number and range of communities of practice vary throughout life, and what is learnt from these communities is personally transformative.

> ## Reflective activity
>
> Identify all the communities of practice that you belong to currently, and then compare this list to your own situation 10 years ago. Think about how some of the communities of practice you were part of 10 years ago have affected your learning.

Situated learning is what individuals acquire by contributing to communities of practice, and communities continue to learn and refine their practice and to ensure continued membership. Lave and Wenger (1991) refer to an encompassing process called '**legitimate peripheral participation**' which is a defining characteristic of situated learning.

The term legitimate peripheral participation could, for example, relate to the experience of a student occupational therapist who is a 'newcomer'; in this context, the student's clinical supervisor could be viewed as an 'old-timer'. As time goes on, members of a community of practice start to understand the instances when 'old-timers' collaborate, collide and collude and also what is enjoyed, disliked, respected and admired in the group. Novices participate partially in examples of practice where these values are displayed. Over time, their depth of involvement grows and they redefine their identity. Novices learn actions, and a holistic explanation, from practitioners in the 'real world' setting and this helps them to handle some of the problems relating to the transference of learning.

It is suggested that nursing knowledge acquired in the authentic context has a better chance of being activated when needed in another situation (Lauder *et al.*, 1999). Looking at learning as being situated and encompassed within communities of practice does not mean that telling students to 'go out into practice' or just letting them loose into a clinical area is appropriate.

⚷ Keywords

Legitimate peripheral participation

Legitimate peripheral participation is the process of increasing membership of a community of practice. It is legitimate because the learner is accepted as a potential community member working on the periphery of the community and acquiring knowledge through their practice with 'old-timers'. Learning occurs through the process of becoming a full participant

> ## Reflective activity
>
> Think about the first day that you went into your current or most recent practice setting. What things would you have like to have known sooner, or been told about before you went into this clinical area?

You may have identified a number of things that you learnt through practice that with hindsight you would like to have been told by a mentor or colleague. However, it does not really work if you try to tell newcomers to a clinical area everything you think they will need, as many things cannot be put into words but are learnt through doing. In the following excerpt from an interview, a mentor talks about how she learnt through practice to support students.

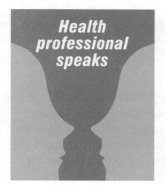

Health professional speaks

Mentor

The mentorship preparation programme was disappointing, although reflecting on how you teach was good. I felt I learnt more from teaching the students in the ward setting. I like to have more practical advice, and I believe that you can learn from everybody, and you need to try and be open to that at home and work.

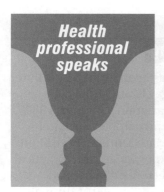

🔑 Keywords

Communal memory

Communal memory involves the recollections and stories of past times and events that continue to be referred to by a community of people

Health care settings can be stressful environments, and communities of practice can help staff to invent and maintain ways of coping. Wenger (1998) suggests that this can be accomplished through the resolution of conflict, reference to a **communal memory**, helping 'newcomers' to join, and determining 'what needs to be done'.

Communities of practice help in the management of difficult situations, such as high workload or interprofessional conflict. In the following excerpt, an operating department practitioner (ODP) talks about how things have changed within their professional learning and the impact on multidisciplinary working.

Health professional speaks

Operating department practitioner

I think ODPs are changing for the better. It's nice to see us being given the opportunity to go and do further degrees; if we want to, it's there. It gives the theatre staff more credibility and allows us to stand our ground with doctors if we don't agree.

In the previous excerpt, an ODP indicates that there is often a level of conflict between the theatre-based staff and the surgeons. Although a community of practice sounds like it would be a site of harmony, it is understandable that within any group there will be multiple viewpoints.

Reflective activity

Think about the last three months and your working in a practice area over this time. How much of your learning was the consequence of time spent with a mentor/clinical supervisor, and how much was the consequence of working with a range of staff within your clinical setting?

Communities of practice can serve as a 'living repository of knowledge', knowledge that can be 'sticky and leaky' and cross boundaries (Wenger *et al.*, 2002, p. 153). When you were reflecting on the past three months, some of your learning may well have been difficult to identify either in your thoughts or in writing, but you could perhaps have talked about it more easily with another person. The tacit aspects of knowledge are often the most valuable and can be shared through storytelling, conversation, coaching and learner support.

Key points Top tips

- Individuals and communities learn through their everyday practice
- Legitimate peripheral participation is the process whereby novices progress towards full membership of a community of practice
- Communities of practice are forums for situated knowledge, and can assist in resolving conflict

Professional knowledge and learning

Understanding about professional knowledge has been limited by failure to conceptualise the different types of knowledge (Eraut, 1994). A professional is able to recognise 'situation and variation' (Benner, 1984), make competent judgements in unpredictable and complex situations, and apply knowledge and skills with the appropriate attitudes. Oakshott (1962) makes a distinction between 'technical knowledge' and 'practical knowledge'. Technical knowledge is written and codified, whereas practical knowledge is expressed only in practice and is learnt through experience in practice settings. Patel *et al.* (1999) suggest that there are two types of knowledge, factual knowledge that can be verbalised and intuitive knowledge that cannot. People acquire personal knowledge through experiences, either directly or vicariously. Personal knowledge is constructed through interaction with the wider context in which the experience occurs. In practice settings, all of these forms of knowledge are inextricably linked as a 'dynamic, integrated whole' (Williams, 1998, p. 28).

Over to you

Read: Hall, V. and Hart, A. (2004) The use of imagination in professional education to enable learning about disadvantaged clients. *Learning in Health and Social Care*, **3**(4), 190–202.

The sort of ideas expressed in the previous article question the traditional view of professional knowledge in which propositional knowledge gained from lectures and texts has to be reconstructed and applied in practice settings. Situated learning implies that knowledge and mastery of skills can only be acquired and successfully retained through practice in social, workplace contexts which are developing, changing and modifying. This rejects the separation of learning and the application of learning. If it is accepted that knowing is primarily about participating in a community of practice, then educational resources need to be directed at inventive ways of engaging students in meaningful practices, such as involving students in actions, discussions and reflections.

Reflective activity

Think about your local educational institute. In what ways do the staff and structures you know of reflect a movement towards action-based learning, discussion and reflective activities?

Practitioners should look critically at their own practice as part of their everyday routine, but they often seek to justify their practice rather than analyse it. The learner may well be able to view 'professional artistry' in action, but probably finds it more difficult to get to discuss what underpins this with a mentor or supervisor. Reflection can be a process for making explicit professionals' practical knowledge, and learners can process, interpret and generalise from their own experience and create mental frameworks to aid their understanding (Harrison *et al.*, 2002).

Situated learning is based on 'professional artistry', where only the principles or frameworks can be pre-determined and practitioners may for good 'context-specific' reasons choose to go beyond these principles (Fish and Coles, 1998). Schön (1983) discusses the importance of artistry within professional practice and questions the '**technical rationality**' model of professional knowledge as only applying to simplified problems and not the complex problems faced by professional practitioners.

The so called 'theory–practice gap' is seen as an artefact of the technical–rational view of professional education and can only exist where there is a belief that there is a clear separation of theoretical knowledge from practical knowledge (Fish and Coles, 1998, p. 45). Schön identified reflection-in-action, which occurs at the time of the encounter, and involves looking at our experience connecting with feelings and tacit knowledge, and reflection-on-action which occurs later after the encounter. Eraut (1994) is critical of Schön's (1983) notion of reflection-in-action, suggesting that it is really not reflection at all, but a single 'gut' judgement working in a reflexive rather than reflective fashion. Situated learning suggests that those who 'facilitate', 'coach' and 'mentor' have more relevance than those who purely 'teach' (Harrison *et al.*, 2002). There is also increased significance in informal learning gained through social relationships with colleagues, mentors, line managers and specialists (Eraut *et al.*, 1998).

Researchers who have focused on the importance of situated learning within nursing have mainly looked at this in relation to student nurses (Burkitt *et al.*, 2000; Cope *et al.*, 2000). Pre-registration student nurses talked about 'earning' social and professional acceptance which was not helped by short-duration placements (Cope *et al.*, 2000). Burkitt *et al.* (2000) identified two major problems facing student nurses: their location was within two communities of practice (higher education institute and clinical placements) and there were insufficiently strong links between the two. The multi-levelled nature of knowledge and practice needs to be reflected in the nursing curriculum through increased nurse lecturer involvement in practice and enhanced support for mentors (Burkitt *et al.*, 2000). At present, the multiple roles and multiple demands placed on experienced nurses leads to a process of successive interruptions and this, when combined with the fragmentation of practice placements and modularisation, can reduce the meaningful learning opportunities for student nurses.

○—ᴙ *Keywords*

Technical rationality
Technical rationality views professional knowledge as being about empirical and scientific forms of evidence-based practice

Community of practice development

There is no doubt that the clinical milieu is full of rich learning experiences, and that learning is more meaningful if the student participates actively within a clinical team whilst on placement. Six factors have been identified as playing key roles: staff (registered and assistants)–student relationships, the manager, commitment to teaching, patient relationships, student satisfaction and hierarchy/ritual (Dunn and Hansford, 1997). Pearcey and Elliott (2004) found that the culture of the clinical area impacted both on the student learning experience and also on their impressions of their chosen profession. It is more than just the availability of time that imparts a caring, better culture: the whole philosophy of the clinical team affected the atmosphere (Pearcey and Elliott, 2004).

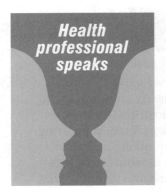

Health professional speaks

Third-year student

It is really refreshing to be on a placement where there is good morale and they're well staffed. When the team aren't particularly negative and are happy about their care delivery, it can make a difference to whether you want to stay on the course and qualify. My experience on this placement has made me change my mind about carrying on to work in this field when I qualify.

Community-building skills are displayed through practitioners' warmth and concern for others and the ambience of an active community. One of the most important features of any workplace or community context is the people with whom one interacts – colleagues, friends, customers, clients and acquaintances. An important way, therefore, of improving clinical learning is through investing time and energy into developing team relationships, sharing common objectives and needs to be fulfilled. A range of factors has been found to help in the development of clinical teams and the increasing movement towards group needs. These include:

- personal commitment
- sharing a common goal
- clarity of roles
- good lines of communication
- institutional support
- leadership (Wigens, 2005).

The clinical/ward manager plays a vital role; Smith's (1992) research described the ward sister/charge nurse as the 'architect' of nursing work who sets the emotional and organisational agenda of the ward. A clinical leader in one case study identified how important her own and other staff's CPD had been in influencing improvements in her clinical area (Wigens, 2004). Clinical leadership is linked to a commitment to CPD and lifelong learning, and senior staff acted as role models for this.

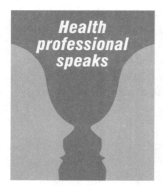

Health professional speaks

Staff nurse – Day Surgery Unit

In our unit here we're given a lot of opportunity to do things because we've got a really good sister who makes sure that we are keeping ourselves up to date. You feel that you want to, because she studies too.

In health care, emphasis has been placed on developing 'transformational leadership', which involves paying attention to the needs of individuals and the group processes, ensuring feedback on performance, developing a stable and trusting workforce, supporting networking and technology and using emotional intelligence (McCormack *et al.*, 2002). Transformational leadership transposes individual beliefs and values into collective beliefs and values so that they become taken for granted. Stordeur *et al.* (2001) suggest that nurses who experience an imbalance between efforts expended at work and the reward obtained are more likely to be emotionally exhausted, and that leadership roles can buffer the effects of a demanding work environment by maintaining a supportive leadership style. Transformational leaders motivate staff to do more than initially expected and are change agents that transmit a sense of mission, instil faith and respect and treat each employee as an individual (Stordeur *et al.*, 2001).

Situational leadership is based on the assumption that there is no one singularly successful leadership style, and that a variety of effective leadership styles should be used, dependent on the context. Some of the skills identified for being an effective facilitator or leader include being a source of clinical advice, having local credibility and understanding of the 'system', and being pragmatic and motivated (Harvey *et al.*, 2002).

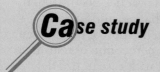

Clinical leadership and its impact on learning

Sian, a community midwife, identified that many teenage women in her clinical locality were not attending antenatal classes regularly, and so did not receive proper care or midwifery support. When Sian discussed this with the community midwifery team, they agreed that this was a priority area to be tackled and also that, as well as accessing these expectant mothers more actively and offering antenatal support in a different way to capture this group, they should work with other stakeholders. Sian set up a group to work on improving antenatal care for teenage mothers, involving user representation, staff from mainstream education, local colleges, adult education centre, Brook advisory centre, health visitors, school nurses and youth services. The group decided that they wanted to work on a way to help teenagers who were pregnant make healthy informed choices about their lifestyle, and therefore their babies' health (e.g. low birthweight is indicative of a tendency to coronary disease in later life, DoH, 2000a). The stakeholders and the midwifery clinical team developed a local resource pack for teenage mothers and a guidance tool for education and health care professionals to use with this antenatal group.

When the midwifery clinical team talked about Sian they described her in the following ways:

- She's inspirational and motivational – she just 'goes for it'.
- She holds on to her vision, even when times get tough, and you can always count on her to do 'the right thing'.
- She is able to listen to other people's views, and to work across boundaries to build relationships.

Having looked at this particular case, can you identify any other things you might add to describe this successful leader?

Have you come across a clinical leader like this within your practice, and did their leadership skills have an impact on the clinical learning environment?

Although the midwife in the previous case study did refer to research findings, her decision-making was not just based on this. The knowledge developed by individual health care practitioners through their decision-making and experience is different from contemporary published scientific knowledge. Networking can involve sharing of knowledge through person-to-person contact, and oral story telling, which is particularly well developed in health care, can be a way of communicating knowledge, as practitioners find it easier to talk about good practice, rather than write about it (Burke and Smith, 2000).

Practitioners do not apply research findings in a simple deductive process: they need time to think, translate and particularise research findings (Titchen, 2000). Competent nurses require 'situational flexibility' and sensitivity to the subtle differences between broadly similar situations, so that they can actively respond in appropriate ways (Phillips *et al.*, 2000a, p. 101). Situated understanding promotes making judgements within complex situations, drawing on tacit and experiential knowledge built up over time. Practice is a relational concept, not an abstract theoretical finding.

Successful implementation of evidence-based practice occurs when the evidence is robust, the context receptive to change, and there is appropriate monitoring, strong leadership and facilitation of the change (Harvey *et al.*, 2002). Timing is important to the perception of relevance, as are professional involvement and engagement with research. The extent to which a given piece of evidence is utilised by an individual in practice depends on their sense of the situation and inevitably involves professional judgement. Within medicine, this application of research findings to the demands of everyday practice has been termed 'context-sensitive medicine' (Greenhalgh and Worrall, 1997). Further examination of practice development is included in Chapter 7.

Strategies for making non-research knowledge explicit include reflection, discussion of critical incidents in the clinical setting, enhancement of evaluative cultures, peer review, and clinical supervision (LeMay, 1999). Making time for staff discussions about the effectiveness of clinical practice and clinical supervision/mentorship within the setting could address concerns and lead to continual improvement.

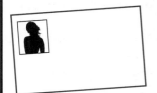

Clinical Caseload . . .

At a ward staff meeting, the following suggestions were made for improving the quality of clinical learning experiences for qualified practitioners and students (adapted from Palmer *et al.*, 2005, Table 2).

1   Students need to undertake complete care interventions for their patients, as much as is feasible given their skills level.

2   All staff should be provided with information on the current skill level of students and their learning objectives for the clinical area.

3   Students should work the same shift pattern and attend all clinical team discussions, so that they are integrated members of the health care delivery team.

4   All mentors/supervisors should be provided with information on how to effectively mentor students and new staff to the area.

Do you agree with the suggestions? Would you add any further suggestions to be discussed in the staff meeting?

Learning organisations should pay attention to the needs of individuals and groups as well as to the organisational systems. Wenger and colleagues' (2002) exploration of communities of practice relationships to their employing organisation identified five main relationships:

1 unrecognised or invisible

2 bootlegged, and only visible informally to the circle of people in the know

3 legitimised and officially sanctioned as valuable

4 strategic and widely recognised as central to organisational success

5 transformative, and capable of redefining its environment.

As clinical teams develop, they may progress through these levels of relationships within their institutions. What level would you choose to describe the ward team who attended the staff meeting in the previous clinical caseload?

A hidden curriculum of observed behaviour and interactions and the overall norms and culture of a student's training environments shape the values, attitudes and professional identity of future health care professionals. Professional identity is integrated with a personal sense of identity and involves the individual's having a feeling of being able to practise with skill, being able to articulate clearly their commitment to their profession, and taking responsibility for their own actions, whilst maintaining an awareness of their attributes and limitations (Ohlen and Segesten, 1998).

As individuals are members of many communities of practice, identity can be multi-dimensional and arises in interaction with others (Sarup, 1996). Situated learning is personally meaningful. Motivation, activity and learning are related to positive self-esteem and identity, and the individual health care practitioner is shaped by their relationship to their community of practice. For example, membership of a nursing community is inextricably linked with individual motivations to nurse and engagement through development of a 'professional identity'. This 'professional identity' motivates learning and working and is not always 'switched off' when a nurse leaves work (Wigens, 2004). Although there is a sense of being a member of a 'common nursing profession', over time the nurse also becomes aligned to the health care context. There is internalisation of the values, knowledge, skills, norms and culture occurring in relation to nursing, but also towards the speciality in which the nurse works.

My own research found that nurses saw their work in their speciality as clearly different from other areas of nursing and were keen to ensure that their speciality was recognised as different from others (Wigens, 2004). Within the hospital, nurses aligned themselves very easily to medically defined specialities: e.g. surgical nurses in line with the speciality of the surgical consultants who related to these ward areas. This is perhaps unsurprising as the domination of biomedicine is felt to be strongest in hospital settings, and there is a general acceptance that specialisation attempts to improve the quality of care.

Nurses were clear about what is attractive about their speciality, in comparison with other areas of nursing, and conscious of how the perceived 'image' of their nursing speciality was currently constructed and affected things such as recruitment of staff (Wigens, 2004). It was interesting to note that nurses' accounts of what they preferred about their speciality were often used as a reason by another nurse to discount the choice of that speciality for themselves. These descriptors of their specialisms tended to relate to the type of client and the length of the client–nurse relationship. Examples of their reasons for enjoying/preferring their specialities are outlined in Table 4.2.

Being able to outline the differences between the chosen speciality and the professional role to others is part of nurses' striving for positive social identity. Membership of groups, cliques and sub-groups within the nursing workplace is valuable both for mutual support and help, and it also increases power, allowing nurses to gain control and resist unwanted change. Nurses consider reflective discussions with colleagues during group supervision as important in the development of their professional identity and for community building (Ohlen and Segesten, 1998).

Key points Top tips

- Clinical learning is most effective within a clinical milieu where practitioners are engaged, warm, reflective and work together with active concern for staff and patients
- It is worth investing time and energy in the development of a community of practice, including its knowledge base
- Transforming situational leadership is vital in ensuring effective clinical learning opportunities
- Communities of practice influence the professional identities of both qualified practitioners and students

Table 4.2 Nurses' descriptions of their speciality – client type and length of stay (Wigens, 2004)

Speciality	Client type	Length of stay
Medical Nursing	'There's usually more than one problem, and it's complicated.' '[It's] a sort of balancing juggling act.'	'You get more social problems so it takes a while to arrange discharges, although the length of stay has reduced. We no longer get convalescing patients.'
Accident and Emergency Nursing	'I like the variety of patients; there's not just one speciality; it ranges from paediatrics through to care of the elderly . . . and of course the adrenalin buzzes with multiple traumas.'	'There's always something different. New faces every day. Every half an hour the workload is different. From minor to major and back to minor again.'
Care of the Elderly Nursing	'I usually like the people on care of the elderly and find it rewarding. I like the social aspects; you're more involved, and care seems more complete.'	'We get time to know the patients a bit more. For example we can have two days off and there's more or less the same patients when we return.'
District Nursing	'I like the variety of work, terminal care, palliative care, wound management, diabetic care – basically anything.' 'The nicest part for me is seeing people in their own homes as part of a family, community.'	'It's real life. We see the end of the story. I've got people on my caseload that I've known since I started district nursing. They'll be there until I leave or they die. So you've got continuity.'
Surgical Nursing	'I enjoy nursing the major surgical cases best, where the patient is acutely ill and we work to get them discharged.' 'It's good when you have a variety of operations.'	'I like the fast patient turnover – seeing the patient come into hospital and recover quickly so that they can go home.'
Day Surgery Nursing	'The outcomes are generally positive, clients are fit and well and it's rewarding to see the patient "cured".'	'You're able to see the patient through from admission to discharge – following the whole patient episode.'

Possible problems within communities of practice

Within any community of practice there is a risk that innovators will be 'held hostage' to the experience of the 'elders', with statements such as, 'We've tried that before and it didn't work' (Wenger, 1998, p. 85). Because of this, a community of practice can become so insular that its members become unable to register other viewpoints, and this can become an obstacle to learning and change (Wenger, 1998, p. 98). Members of a community of practice, like any social group, can specialise, gain reputation, distinguish, create different statuses, join cliques and share gossip. Enthusiasm can lead to arrogance, and a community can become dependent on one leader. Alternatively, a community can become marginalised and not be taken seriously (Wenger et al, 2002).

In leaving professional learning totally to 'legitimate peripheral participation' there is a possibility that practice could become outmoded, inherited from 'old-timers' with a lack of new ideas to stimulate changes in practice. Lave and Wenger (1991) argue that stagnation will not occur, however, because the focus of learning continues through the 'community of practice' and knowledge is continuously created.

Reflective activity

Have you ever been in a clinical setting and felt that practice had become outmoded and was stagnating? What factors did you feel had the most impact on this situation?

An under-developed aspect of Lave and Wenger's (1991) theory of situated learning is the role given to reflection on practice (Maudsley and Strivens, 2000), and it would be a good idea to link your understanding of communities of practice to the discussion on reflection incorporated in Chapter 7. Although Lave and Wenger (1991, p. 109) identify 'talking about' practice and relating stories as a form of memory and reflection, they say little about the way that stories are regularly revised to take account of changing needs, aspirations and motivations.

Some critics claim that Lave and Wenger's theory is too all-encompassing, with its assertion that all learning takes place within the social setting, and argue for a distinction between social learning and individual learning, with individual learning taking place independently of the social context. It is alleged that one risk in over-advocating the value of situated learning is that it undermines the role of professional education that is delivered within educational institutes with the expectation that this will be transferred to practice. Perhaps the problem is that some interpretations of Lave and Wenger's work have incorrectly concluded that they are claiming that knowledge learnt in a classroom setting cannot be used in practice. My view is that the social and individual are so intertwined that you cannot just focus on the individual. The individual aspects of clinical learning are explored within the next chapter.

Key points ~~Top tips~~

- There is a risk with communities of practice that they can become insular, marginalised and less open to change
- The concept of communities of practice needs to be further developed with regard to the role of reflection and frameworks for participation

RRRRRRapid recap

Check your progress so far by working through each of the following questions.

1   What types of student–patient relationship may be developed within a clinical learning environment?

2   Define the 'hidden curriculum' within health care professional education.

3   What, in the view of Weidman *et al.* (2001), are the four components of professional socialisation?

4   Explain in your own words the following concepts:
    (a) legitimate peripheral participation
    (b) communal memory
    (c) professional artistry.

5   Identify five factors that help the development of a community of practice clinical team.

6   List three possible problems with relying on community of practice processes for clinical learning.

If you have difficulty with one of these questions, read through the section again to refresh your understanding before moving on.

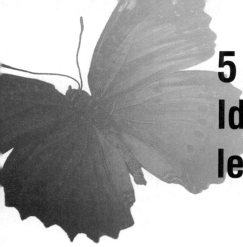

5
Identifying individual learning needs

Learning outcomes

By the end of this chapter you should be able to:

★ Explain the factors that affect your learning

★ Undertake an assessment of your learning style

★ Appreciate the need to balance individual learning needs with job/role requirements

★ Discuss the structure and process of developing a learning contract or a personal development plan.

Introduction

In this chapter, we focus on individual learning. You will think about individual learning stories and the factors that affect these, such as learning styles and motivation. We will also look at how individual learning needs (knowledge and skills) can be identified, objectives set and a plan carried out. As many students and qualified health care practitioners work within the NHS, I have included a brief overview of the Knowledge and Skills Framework, which is now used throughout the NHS, and shown how this can be integrated into an individual learning contract.

Individual learning stories

The best way to start thinking about the individual learner's needs is to consider past learning experiences. When we meet someone for the first time, we often exchange information about where we work and about our family and friends so that we learn something about each other, even though this is usually on quite a superficial level and only gives a small insight into the person. Examining personal learning stories can be a much more illuminating process. Telling one's story can be transformative (Sarup, 1996). When a learner feels comfortable talking about their story, they can illuminate important points about learning preferences and 'blindspots'. This is useful for the mentor as both the learner and their mentor can take into account the different learning histories that participants bring with them.

Reflective activity

Draw a line on a blank sheet of paper, starting with you at age five and continuing to the present day. At various points on this line, identify where you felt your learning experience was significant. For instance, this may be when you first started your health care professional qualification. When you place a point on the line, jot down why there was a 'ramping up' of learning at that time. Then reflect on what this has told you about your 'learning story'.

Health care careers are often explained through mileposts that include a mix of job changes and personal family events. The sense of career capital created by professional qualifications, a career structure and occupational identity means that nurses often return to work following a break for personal, such as family, reasons. However, student nurses are socialised not to bring their 'family issues' to work but to deal sequentially with the demands of work and family role, using a calm, detached coping style (Shiu, 1998). Nurses who leave the profession are viewed as being unable to manage the stress arising from the home–work interface (Shiu, 1998). When people talk about the influences on their lives, they often use the metaphor of a journey in which certain key decisions and experiences determine its route thereafter. Many career decisions are felt to be opportunistic and affected by chance (Wigens, 2004). Looking back on the last reflective activity, you may have felt that it helped to 'flesh out' your learning journey.

Decisions affecting whether you start your health care course, or perhaps choose not to commence a course at another time, are likely to be linked to your home or personal circumstances (Smith and Topping, 2001; Wigens, 2004).

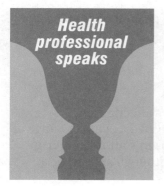

Health professional speaks

Staff nurse – Accident and Emergency Department

Where I worked before, courses were unheard of. Managers didn't push you to do the mentorship preparation course. More recently, courses have become much more available. It's very good; there's so much out there. I've done the mentorship module, started on my degree; I did the counselling module and the research. Then I became pregnant and I haven't picked it up again. My family life is very important: I don't want to leave my little girl. The courses made me think about how I do things, especially when I was doing my counselling and afterwards.

Working in an area that makes it possible to access post-registration courses increases individual learning opportunities. Success in pre- and post-registration studies appear to be linked to the motivation and hard work of the student, their personal life situation, and the support given by the employer in terms of funding or study leave. Nurses talk about critical incidents or informal social/group interactions within their career that act as catalysts to their professional learning (Wigens, 2004). Individual motivators to learn, knowledge of oneself as a learner, and a disposition to learn, as well as service area benefits, are seen as the key to successful continuous professional development (CPD), and successful personal development plans are negotiated with all these elements in mind.

The following case study account is from a staff nurse working in an Accident and Emergency department; it identifies many of the factors that are linked to lifelong learning in nursing. Read the account and identify key factors that affected this staff nurse's individual lifelong learning.

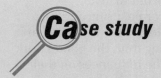

Factors affecting lifelong learning

I was just plodding along, getting sluggish and fed up with nursing. The conversion course helped because as an enrolled nurse I couldn't go any further. I know I was very close to leaving nursing if I hadn't got on the conversion course. I'm a lot happier now I can do more things, like plastering, and I wouldn't have been able to do an A & E course as an enrolled nurse. The modules I've been doing on the A & E course make me see how little I know about certain things. I know a little bit about most things and I use the profiles to increase my knowledge.

The course has highlighted what I want to go on and find out a bit more about. Things that go on in the department mean that I want to learn more about certain things. The conversion course wasn't what I was expecting; I was hoping to learn more anatomy and physiology. But then I've gone out and done it myself. I see myself as staying in A & E and I'd like to do my Registered Mental Nurse training to use in the department. It's not just the work here that has led to an interest in mental health, but I've had involvement with people close to me with mental health problems in my personal life. I'm also told that I'm very good with the suicide patients. I find time to talk to them, and a lot of the time that's all they want. In my personal life I've had a lot of things to cope with from a very young age and that's made me, I think, a very strong person anyway.

From reading the previous account of the factors affecting an individual's lifelong learning, you will have identified a complex range of interrelated aspects. You probably also noted this in your reflection on your own lifelong learning. Self-development, although appearing individual, is also social in nature.

Individual continuous professional development

There is a long history of researchers studying the CPD activities of professionals: for example, Mackereth (1989) and Smith and Topping (2001). Ryan (2003) found no difference in motivational factors between nurses, occupational therapists and physiotherapists; increasing professional knowledge and competence was the most common reason for undertaking CPD. The need for CPD has been heightened by the realisation that a professional's claim to possess specific, advanced knowledge can only be made in the light of evidence that professional education is ongoing and effective. Organisational and managerial reforms demand that practitioners be self-motivated regarding their personal and professional development.

Fox *et al.* (1989) suggest that the motivation to change aspects of practice is most often rooted in a passion to do a better job, not out of feeling incompetent but from a desire to be as competent as individuals can be with regard to their practice. Within one case site, the outcome of engaging in CPD was assessed in terms of both the visible changes in an individual's nursing practice and CPD's ability to develop careers by preparing nurses for promotion (Wigens, 2004). It can be difficult to determine the full impact of individual CPD activities on health care practice as the development of the individual is inextricably linked with their own personal development and clinical/professional development. Individual motivations are explored in the next section.

Motivation

The concept of motivation seems to provide an answer to the question, 'What makes us do the things we do?' Motivation is what leads us to behave, act or learn in specific, purposeful ways. One of the pioneers of motivation research, Cyril Houle (1961), identified three categories of adult learner:

- goal-oriented (pursuing identified objectives)
- learning-oriented (learning for the love of it)
- activity-oriented (learning for reasons unconnected with objectives but task related).

These categories are still largely accepted although it is now common to reduce them to a simple dichotomy – learning for instrumental motives (to achieve specific goals) or for intrinsic motives (learning for its own sake). However, this instrumental-versus-intrinsic division is perhaps too simplistic as people often have mixed motives for learning. One could focus on individual characteristics, such as learning styles and motivation, or on 'attractors' and 'deterrents' affecting participation in continuing education activities, assessing the role that workplace challenges and opportunities play in individuals' learning activities.

Maslow (1954) defined a hierarchy of needs that should be satisfied before effective learning can occur. He suggested that these needs must be attended to in their hierarchical order. They are:

- physiological – to be fed and watered
- safety – freedom from excessive anxiety
- social – the need to be loved and cared for, respected as a person
- self-esteem – skills mastered; recognition by others
- self-fulfilment – personal achievement, freedom to take responsibility, be creative and develop.

elleR*Reflective activity*

Look at the following quote from a staff nurse on a ward:

> Some of the senior sisters come on and they see you're still there say half-past four, quarter to five and you're still the early shift. I don't think it really sinks in that we're still there and that we're still working when we should have finished at three and we haven't had a lunch break or a coffee break and we're still there.. . . It's a very long day and you know you're not stopping to drink or eat. I've had to make a conscious effort now because I passed out on the ward and it was just because I was just so tired and I wasn't drinking. I hadn't had anything to eat and I was just totally exhausted. I think you really have to make yourself sit down sometimes.

Do you think this nurse's comments have any connection to Maslow's hierarchy of need and its link with motivations to learn? Do any of the factors identified by Maslow affect your motivation to learn in clinical settings? What needs do you think need to be met before clinical learning is likely to occur?

When health care practitioners perceive a need to learn something, they are generally capable of working very hard, but as adults with many roles (e.g. spouse, parent, employee, student) they are often time-conscious learners. Therefore, most want to meet their educational goals as directly, quickly, and efficiently as possible. The challenge is to create a non-threatening atmosphere in which practitioners have permission to learn and are expected to share in the responsibility for their learning. Establishing 'adult-to-adult' rapport and using positive non-verbal and verbal communication can help to create the right atmosphere. The mentor needs to deal with the whole person, addressing the learner as an equal and employing an informally structured approach. Adult learners appreciate supervisors who share appropriate information and are approachable and accessible.

Factors that act as sources of motivation for learning include:

- meeting and making new professional and personal relationships
- complying with external expectations from the higher education institute and the professional bodies
- improving the individual's ability to serve the 'community of practice' or clinical team
- achieving higher status in a job and securing professional advancement
- an escape, or for stimulation, by providing a break in the routine of home or work
- for cognitive interest: to learn for the sake of learning, seeking knowledge for its own sake, and to satisfy an inquiring mind.

How that energy is directed and at what level may be a direct result of the social context of each individual learner. When the presence of a group motivates an individual to pursue a particular behaviour, it is called social facilitation. If the nature of the task or discussion within the group is interesting, interactive and involving, it is more likely to motivate the individual to achieve. This is especially true if the individual feels a personal affinity or particular talent for the task.

Reflective activity

Think about your recent areas of interest and about learning situations where you put in more effort than you needed to. What was it about that particular area of practice learning that motivated you?

We can easily get into 'habits' regarding our learning; habitual action refers to what has been previously learnt and becomes automatic through frequent use. A habit is at the intersection between knowledge, skill and desire (Covey, 1999) and is non-reflective.

* Knowledge is 'what to do and why'.
* Skill is 'how to do'.
* Desire is 'motivation and the want to do'.

Knowledge, skill and desire have to interrelate for effective habits to develop. For example, you may have noted that you are a poor listener regarding peer worker problems. You may know that you need to listen and you may know how to listen, but if you don't have the desire to listen it won't be a habit in your life.

Seven main habits of highly effective people (Covey, 1999)

Habit 1 – Be Proactive
Habit 2 – Begin with the end in mind
Habit 3 – Put first things first
Habit 4 – Think win/win
Habit 5 – Seek first to understand then to be understood
Habit 6 – Synergize
Habit 7 – Sharpen the saw

According to Covey (1999), habits 1, 2 and 3 deal with self-mastery, that is, moving from dependence (you do it) to independence (I do it). These habits are seen as 'private victories', the essence of personal learning and growth: learning to define oneself, rather than relying purely on other people's opinions or by comparison to others. Private victories are viewed as the precursor to public victories. Habits 4, 5 and 6, are personality-oriented 'public victories', involving interdependence (we do it), teamwork, co-operation and communication. These habits foster improved relationships and the desire to rebuild important relationships. Habit 7 is one of renewal, and Covey (1999) suggests that this should encircle all the other habits. A habit of continuous improvement and self-renewal is viewed as creating the upward spiral for growth. Reflecting on, and having an awareness of habits which reduce our ability to learn and that reduce our personal effectiveness, is required.

The length of time that learner motivation can be sustained is variable, hence the usefulness of periodic reviews of progress through, for example, learning contracts or personal development plan review meetings. These not only help the learner to gain understanding of their achievements but also determine what action both the learner and the mentor/supervisor need to take.

Learning styles

Students may become more motivated to learn by knowing more about their own strengths and weaknesses as learners. The issue of learning styles has been partly addressed by the development of learning style models, of which there are many. Coffield *et al.* (2004) looked at 71 models of learning styles and then categorised 13 of these as major models. Within this chapter I have chosen to look at four of these, the last three of which are most commonly used within health care practice.

The four models presented briefly here take varying forms, being based on genetics (Dunn, 2003), personality type (Myers and McCaulley, 1998) and flexible learning preferences (Honey and Mumford, 1992; Kolb, 1984a). Some theorists have strong beliefs about the influence of genetics on fixed, inherited traits and about the interaction of personality and cognition. However, Dunn and Dunn's model (Dunn, 2003) does also acknowledge external factors, such as the immediate environment. Genetics-based models are rooted in ideas that styles should be worked with rather than changed. Other models of learning style are based on the relationship between self and experience with some paying greater attention to personal factors such as motivation, and others stressing the importance of environmental factors such as whether learning is collective or individual.

The Dunn and Dunn model

According to this model, a learning style is divided into five main elements that significantly influence what individuals learn; these are called stimuli. The stimulus elements are:

- environmental
- emotional
- sociological
- psychological
- physiological (Dunn, 2003, p. 2).

From these elements certain factors are thought to affect students' preferences (see Table 5.1, adapted from Coffield *et al.*, 2004).

Table 5.1 Factors affecting learning

Element	Factors			
Environmental	Sound	Temperature	Light	Clinical area layout
Psychological	Likes to learn alone	Likes to learn in pairs	Likes to learn in a group	Likes to learn as part of a team
Emotional	Motivation	Need for structure	Degree of responsibility	Persistence
Physiological	Modality preference for VAKT[1] • Visual • Auditory • Kinaesthetic/ Tactile	Physical functioning e.g. intake (food and drink)	Time of day	Mobility
Sociological	Learning group	Help and support from authority figures, e.g. mentor/ supervisor	Working alone or with peers	Motivation of the educator

[1]VAKT modalities are explained in the next section of this chapter.

The Dunn and Dunn model places a strong emphasis on biological and developmentally imposed characteristics. Each person's unique combination of preferences comprises their learning style. People who have no high or low preferences do not need 'matching' and can therefore adapt more easily to different learning activities. The model measures preferences rather than strengths and takes the view that we should not stigmatise different types of preference.

VAKT modalities

For effective learning to occur, a learner needs to feel comfortable with the methods used. Individuals can develop a preference for sending and receiving information through one sense over another. People more commonly prefer auditory or visual input; however, some people have a preference for kinaesthetic/tactile learning: learning that involves movement or touch. A preference for one type of learning over another can be identified.

- Visual learners prefer or enjoy graphic illustrations such as bar graphs to explain data; colour coding to highlight salient information; flowcharts within clinical guidelines; written material; wall charts that display points to be remembered; written outlines; drawings or designs to illustrate overhead presentations; looking at gestures or visuals.

- Auditory learners prefer or enjoy verbal presentation of new information; group discussions; fast-paced verbal exchanges of ideas; a good joke or story; verbal cues or mnemonic devices to help them remember information (e.g. ABC for Airway, Breathing, Circulation); oral reports of working.

- Kinesthetic/tactile learners prefer or enjoy movement such as hands-on experience to learn a task; gesturing whilst making a point; role-play exercises; shaking hands when meeting or greeting people; trying new things without a lengthy explanation of the activity; frequent breaks; 'just doing it' rather than talking about it.

While it is thought that people have developed a preference for or have greater skill in processing one type of input over others, for most people information is processed simultaneously through multiple senses. In fact, the retention of learnt material is enhanced if the learner is able to use all senses.

> ## Over to you
>
> Identify your preferred learning modality. There are a number of tests available on line that you could try: for example, go to www.businessballs.com and select the learning styles VAK test.

The Myers-Briggs Type Indicator

The Myers-Briggs Type Indicator (MBTI) was developed in the early 1940s with the aim of making Jung's theory of human personality understandable and useful in everyday life (Myers and McCaulley 1998). The MBTI looks at the descriptions of normally observed types based on personality factors.

The four bipolar scales of the MBTI are:

Extraversion (E) ———————— Introversion (I)
Sensing (S) ———————— Intuition (N)
Thinking (T) ———————— Feeling (F)
Judging (J) ———————— Perceiving (P)

From these 8 personality features were developed 16 MBTI personality types: for example, ENTP (Extraversion, Intuition, Thinking, Perceiving).

Over to you

There are a range of on-line tools adapted from the MBTI that you could try. You can read more about Myers-Briggs personality types by looking at the section titled 'Myers-Briggs personality theory and MBTI types indicator' at www.businessballs.com.

Do you agree with the findings, and what the type identified for you says?

Kolb's Learning Styles Inventory

The Learning Styles Inventory (LSI) was developed by David Kolb in the early 1970s and linked his theory of experiential learning to an instrument devised both to test his theory and to capture individual learning differences (Kolb, 1984a). He observed that some students had definite preferences for some activities: for example, some liked exercises but others preferred lectures. For Kolb (1984a), a learning style is not a fixed trait but a differential preference for learning, which changes slightly from situation to situation. However, he acknowledges that there is some longer-term stability in learning style. Kolb's four dominant learning styles are each located in a different quadrant of the cycle of experiential learning.

The learning cycle stages are:

1 concrete experience – feeling – having the experience
2 reflective observation – watching – reviewing the experience
3 abstract conceptualisation – thinking – concluding from the experience
4 active experimentation – doing – planning the next stage.

The four learning styles within Kolb's LSI are:

- **diverging** (concrete experience and reflective observation) – imaginative, interested in people, breadth of interests
- **assimilating** (abstract conceptualisation and reflective observation) – theory creator, uses reasoning, able to handle abstract concepts

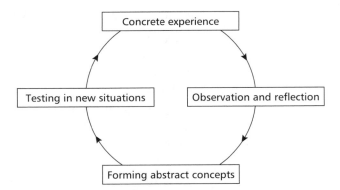

Figure 5.1 Diagram of Kolb's experiential learning cycle (after Kurt Lewin, 1942)

- **converging** (abstract conceptualisation and active experimentation) – application to practice, depth of interest
- **accommodating** (concrete experience and active experimentation) – does things and takes risks, uses intuition to solve problems.

Kolb claimed that an appreciation of differing learning styles helps people to work more effectively in teams, resolve conflict, communicate at work and at home, and choose careers.

Over to you

Take a look at Chapter 2, pages 10–15 in Pearce, R. (2003) Foundations in Nursing and Health Care. *Profiles and Portfolios of Evidence*. Nelson Thornes, Cheltenham.

Identify your learning style using Kolb's LSI and think about how useful this could be to your learning in the future.

Kolb (1984a) suggests that his theory of experiential learning provides a useful framework for the design and management of all learning experiences by encouraging facilitators of learning to provide explicitly for the differences in individual learning styles. For example, the students scoring highest in active experimentation are helped in their learning by small-group discussions, projects, peer feedback and homework, but less so by lectures.

Reflective activity

Think about what learning approaches might be more successful within a clinical setting for each of the four learning style 'types'. Do you foresee any difficulties in a mentor/supervisor adapting negotiation of a learning contract to 'fit' with the individual learning preferences?

Honey and Mumford's (1992) Learning Styles

Honey and Mumford (1992) acknowledged their intellectual debt to Kolb's (1984a) theory, but decided to produce their own learning style questionnaire and to change the unwieldy terms. They changed:

- diverger to reflector
- assimilator to theorist
- converger to pragmatist
- accommodator to activist.

Activists are said to have a preference for experiencing something immediately. They don't read the instruction manual first, but get straight on with the job. They want to do as many new things as possible and like short-term goals, often offering to lead. Reflectors prefer to 'wait and see', reviewing experiences or mulling over data. They take time to think before answering a question and can seem uncertain. Theorists like to build systems and to get first principles agreed. They speak in general rather than in concrete terms and draw conclusions in an objective manner. Pragmatists tend to be confident and energetic, taking short cuts and devising new ways of working. They enjoy problem solving and planning the next steps.

As all of these approaches to learning are viewed as useful, it is advocated that learners become proficient in all four. The complete learner would possess the ability to adopt all with equal facility, but there are not many such learners around, and most people have a preferred or dominant learning style, which can be explored by questionnaire (Honey and Mumford, 1992). Rather than ask people directly how they learn, Honey and Mumford designed a questionnaire, which probes general behavioural tendencies rather than learning.

Are the models useful?

Having looked at some of the learning style models and your own learning style, you are probably starting to form an opinion regarding the usefulness to you of this area of educational research. Learning styles have, for some, become an unquestioned part of their professional thinking and practice, allowing a quick and simple way of differentiating students, and this is understandable as the learning style literature promises practitioners a simple solution to the complex problems of improving the attainment, motivation and attitudes of individual students. Others consider these instruments to be unreliable and invalid and potentially damaging, as they may stereotype or label learners, so do not use them in their practice. I believe there is some merit in understanding an individual's learning preferences, but feel that this needs to be integrated into a holistic view of learning through practice.

Individual needs analysis

Adult education views of learning tend to be built on a particular view of 'the self', which we touched upon in Chapter 2 when discussing andragogy. The idea of the adult learner as an autonomous self has become beyond question and the emphasis on learning within professional programmes is often about personal and professional change. Self-directed learning involves learners in finding out on their own initiative what they need to know. Such an active role is more likely to be adopted if the work is appropriately chosen and the learner is encouraged in their learning.

Identifying learning deficits can be difficult, because as health care deliverers we often seek to justify our actions rather than recognise errors or omissions. Everyone who works makes errors and omissions and the ability to acknowledge and work on these should be celebrated. The mentor needs to work with the learner's self-assessment and patient feedback to recognise and act on the areas requiring improvement.

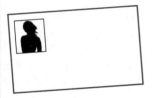

Clinical Caseload . . .

Try using this example of a tool for identifying your learning needs. This activity should be carried out over the course of one shift or working day within clinical practice. Keep a notebook in your pocket and note any unmet patient needs that you recognise – the needs may be unmet because you did not have sufficient skills to deliver this aspect of care or treatment, or you may feel that you could have delivered care in a better way. This activity will enable you to identify an area that would benefit from further learning or development. Areas for learning should be grouped into:

- knowledge (clinical)
- knowledge (non-clinical)
- skill
- attitude.

The second stage involves reflecting on these learning needs with your mentor/ supervisor. These learning needs should be stimulated by the unmet patient needs that you recorded during your clinical working, compiled with other learning needs derived from other sources, such as feedback from patients or colleagues. Your learning needs may be fulfilled in a number of ways, such as by asking an experienced practitioner or by looking up what you need to know; or further study, observation of a specialist practitioner, small group discussion or other forms of learning may be required.

A helpful step is to translate the learning needs into a list of objectives. When you set learning objectives try to make sure they are SMART:

SPECIFIC
MEASURABLE
ACHIEVABLE
REALISTIC
TIMEBOUND.

For example, being asked to 'improve team meetings' is not helpful unless you know how. However, being told to 'ensure all meetings have an agenda, minutes and that you keep to the allotted time' would help because you then know exactly what is expected and whether or not you have achieved the objective.

The following table contains examples of verbs that are useful when formulating objectives. For instance, 'By the end of this clinical placement I will be able to demonstrate. . .'

Table 5.2 Useful verbs

Analyse	Define	Illustrate
Apply	Demonstrate	Interpret
Compare	Differentiate	List
Construct	Explain	Translate
Critique	Identify	Undertake

Reflective activity

Write an individual learning objective based on your current clinical area. Is it SMART? In what ways could you achieve this learning objective? Which learning activity best 'fits' your learning style and the skill, knowledge or attitude to be developed? What forms of evidence can you identify that could be used as the basis for assessing whether this learning outcome had been achieved?

Another way to identify your learning needs could be to undertake a SWOT analysis. A SWOT analysis can be a useful tool not just for identifying individual learning needs but also for examining things that may help or hinder the learning process. You can then try to minimise anything that could impede your learning.

Table 5.3 SWOT pro forma

Strengths	Weaknesses
Opportunities	Threats

Much of your learning is likely to be striving for clinical competence and capability.

Capability involves the integration of confidence in one's ability to take effective and appropriate action, to explain what is being done, to interact effectively with others, and to continue to learn from experiences as an individual and in association with others (Stephenson, 1992).

Competence is the ability to perform a particular activity to a predetermined standard. This predetermined standard can be either:

- criterion referenced – based on a constant reference scale, or
- norm referenced – relating an individual's performance to that of fellow students.

Practitioners need to be able to carry out certain 'tasks' expected by their profession, and health care roles, such as nursing or physiotherapy, call for psychomotor skills as well as analytical and reflective ability. The clinical competence required for work in a practice setting is often well rooted in certain skills, but these also progress and evolve. Acceptable levels of performance influence the assessment of practice processes and also the development of tools by which to judge performance. After developing a learning objective, and agreeing a plan to achieve this, it is necessary to judge whether the learning experience has been effective; where practice skills are concerned, this is usually undertaken through an agreed set of skills criteria.

Skills criteria comprise:

1 a situation of some complexity
2 a performance that deliberately addresses the situation (not just a matter of chance)
3 an assessment that the performance has met the demands of the situation (and is supported by the existence of relevant knowledge)
4 a sense that the performance was commendable.

Undertaking competency-based assessment requires thought, analysis, staff development and effective recording. It can be concerned with what the learner does, rather than what they know, but is best applied with a mechanism that requires understanding of meaning and knowledge. It is helpful if a competency assessment tool, or practice assessment tool, has already been developed and is provided. However, if this is not the case, the learner and supervisor should agree the criteria by which the learning objective is to be judged prior to undertaking the learning activity. There is further exploration of assessment in Chapter 8.

Self-assessment

Self-assessment involves learners taking responsibility for monitoring and making judgements about aspects of their own learning. Although a mentor, supervisor or preceptor may be involved in assessing achievement of a learning objective, it is always useful for the learner to undertake a self-assessment. This can be informal (formative) or formal (summative) in nature and can be broken down into two stages:

1 identifying standards and/or criteria to apply to an understanding of the knowledge, skill or attitude
2 making judgements about the extent to which the learner has met these criteria and standards.

Self-assessment is increasingly being used as a formative tool in clinical education and is frequently used as a means of evaluating learning interventions. However, the ability to assess oneself is seldom tested and self-assessment skills are rarely taught. Self-assessment improves learning by developing the skills of evaluation and critical judgement. In this sense the term 'self-evaluation' may perhaps be more appropriate since, it is about developing learners' ability to make judgements about the quality of their learning.

Self-assessment can:

- help learners to become critical about their own practice
- enable learners to develop their learning and assessment skills whilst engaged in practice rather than afterwards
- provide a structure for discussion about the quality of care/treatment
- help learners to understand the subjective nature of judgements in assessment and the many influences on this.

Reflective activity

Consider whether self-assessment is:

(a) helpful in identifying learning needs
(b) able to promote learner activity
(c) likely to lead to a change in clinical practice.

The NHS Knowledge and Skills Framework

Although individuals have different learner motivations, styles and identified learning needs, it is necessary to appreciate the requirements of a particular health care role. The NHS Knowledge and Skills Framework (KSF) has been designed as a generic development tool for use throughout the NHS to describe the knowledge and skills that are applied within health care and has been designed to support the development of staff (DoH, 2004).

Each post has a KSF outline that identifies the aspects or dimensions of knowledge and skills required for undertaking the role. The KSF is based on 30 dimensions, 6 core dimensions (applied in all roles) and 24 specific dimensions grouped under 4 themes (relevant specifically to the post) as detailed in Table 5.4 below.

Table 5.4 NHS Knowledge and Skills Framework (adapted from DoH, 2004)

Core dimensions:
1. Communication
2. Personal and people development
3. Health, safety and security
4. Service improvement
5. Quality
6. Equality and diversity

Specific dimensions:
Promotion of Health and wellbeing (10 dimensions)

Estates and facilities (3 dimensions)

Information and knowledge (3 dimensions)

General (8 dimensions)

The NHS KSF (DoH, 2004) is designed to:

- support the effective learning and development of individuals and teams – with all staff being supported to learn throughout their careers, and being given the resources to do so
- support the development of individuals in the post in which they are employed so they can be effective at work
- promote equality for and diversity of all staff – with every member of staff using the same framework, having the same opportunities for learning and development open to them and having the same structured approach to learning, development and review.

🔑 Keywords

Appraisal
Appraisal is an organisational process for assessing the performance of staff and their requirement for learning and development. The aim of appraisal is to ensure understanding by staff of what is required of them in their role

✍ Over to you

Take a look at this website, which has been produced to inform everyone about the NHS e-KSF online tool, which supports the Knowledge and Skills Framework:

www.e-ksfnow.org

Progress towards the KSF outline should be reviewed periodically with the employee's line manager. This is usually done within a yearly **appraisal**.

Reflective activity

1   Think about last year – what went well and what not so well? Why was this?
2   What were the most important things that you learnt during the year?
3   Have there been changes in how you give your clinical care?
4   Have you taken on new responsibilities or seen your role change in other ways?

The main elements of an appraisal system are:

- a review of an individual's performance
- identification of training and development needs to ensure full development within an existing post
- supporting and planning career development.

Table 5.5 Roles and responsibilities of appraiser and appraisee

Appraisor	Appraisee
Understand the KSF outline for the posts that you manage or supervise.	Understand the KSF outline for your post.
Undertake appraisal training.	Evaluate your achievements referring to the KSF outline.
Undertake objective reviews of your staff's performance on a regular basis.	Identify your strengths.
Gather and structure evidence to show how members of staff have met their KSF outlines.	Gather and structure evidence that demonstrate your achievements.
Alert staff to issues in their work as soon as they arise.	Identify your learning and development needs.
With the member of staff identify their learning and development needs ensuring that these are included in the post holder's personal development plan.	Prioritise, identify and arrange training and development activities to meet your learning needs.
Identify, with the appraisee, the resources – people, time, finance and equipment – to support their learning.	Identify your personal contribution towards your personal development plan.

Personal development plans

A personal development plan (PDP) is the outcome of a structured support process undertaken by an individual with their manager, to reflect upon their own learning, performance and achievements and to plan for their personal, educational and career development. A PDP is usually agreed through an annual meeting between the individual and their line manager where the performance and progress against the KSF outline are reviewed and new objectives agreed. Following this, there should be ongoing reviews to make sure support and learning is on track. A PDP needs to reflect the changing context of work and an individual's changing knowledge and skills. By agreeing individual objectives within an appraisal, and assessing whether it is necessary to update knowledge or skills, individual development needs are determined.

Prior to the setting up of a PDP, the learner should reflect on their performance and undertake an objective self-assessment. There is often a preparatory form asking you to review your previous year's objectives and personal development plan. It is useful to identify how you can enhance your own contribution and performance in relation to your clinical area's objectives. If you are to have an appraisal and a development or a PDP meeting, you can prepare yourself by answering a few key questions:

1　What have I done well?
2　Where have I been less successful?
3　What obstacles have I met?
4　What important abilities do I have that I am not currently using in my role?
5　What part of my role interests me the most?
6　What part of my role interests me least?
7　Which aspects of my role do I need to gain more experience in or further CPD?
8　Have I undertaken the statutory and mandatory training required this year?
9　In order to help my personal and professional development, what additional things could be done?

Within the meeting you should discuss your individual development and learning needs and those related to your KSF outline. It is also important to follow up the actions agreed during the meeting, especially the learning and development opportunities. Regular conversations with your manager about how your objectives are helping to meet the organisation's aims assist in motivating ongoing learning; these should be linked to regular feedback on your clinical working. It is through individual actions such as these that you can contribute constructively to creating a positive learning environment.

Here is a range of questions to be answered if the PDP is going to be effectively developed:

● What is the development need/interest?
● What will I do to develop myself?
● How will I know I have done this?
● What is the date for planned completion?

- What support do I need and where will I get it?
- What are the barriers and how can I overcome them?
- How will I apply this learning to my work?
- Who else could I share this learning with?

The development objective may be concerned with working towards the level stated in a core or specific KSF dimension for the role, but, as a practitioner develops, the emphasis is likely to shift towards career development. You can use other KSF dimensions to help guide future development if you are looking at different roles in the NHS. Whatever the focus and content of the PDP, it must be agreed between the staff member and the manager. A record of the PDP and associated learning and development can be kept within a Professional Portfolio, along with other CPD documents. Personal development planning should take account of effective learning strategies and connect and draw benefit from reflection (reviewing and evaluating), recording (self-evidencing of learning) and action planning (specific intentions for doing and learning).

Cowan (2002) showed how teachers can learn to improve their own practice through PDP processes (see Figure 5.2).

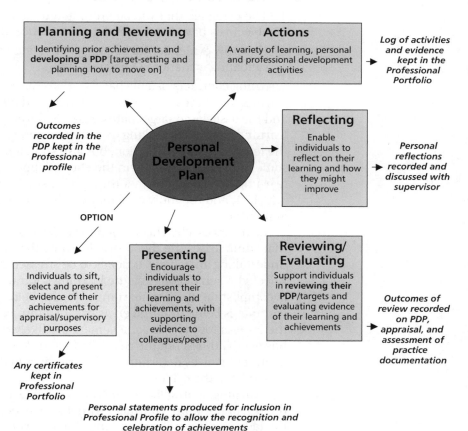

Figure 5.2 Ways in which personal development plans can support individuals in developing their learning (adapted from Cowan, 2002)

Learning contracts

There are many similarities between personal development plans and learning contracts; both are an individualised tool for promoting self-directed adult learning. Essentially, a learning contract is a written plan that describes what an individual will learn as a result of some specified learning activity. Learning contracts can take many forms and a number of terms are used interchangeably in reference to them, such as learning plans, study plans, performance agreements, or self-development plans. Learning contracts can enhance individual motivation for learning and help develop mutual respect between the mentor/supervisor and the learner.

A learning contract consists of five major elements that specify the following:

1 The knowledge, skills, attitudes, and values to be acquired by the learner (learning objectives).

2 How these objectives are to be accomplished by the learner (learning resources and strategies).

3 The target date(s) for completion.

4 The evidence that will be presented to demonstrate that the objectives have been completed (evidence of accomplishment).

5 How this evidence will be judged or validated (criteria and means for validating evidence) (Knowles, 1986).

Learning contracts usually have sections for learning objectives, learning resources, evaluative evidence, and how this will be verified and the associated target dates. A key to developing a successful learning contract is making the learning activities specific enough for the learner to move to action, but also sufficiently flexible to allow some individual creativity in the chosen approach. For instance, a learning need could be met through job shadowing or by participating in a project; and the individual may choose one of these as more appropriate.

Learners can be encouraged to keep a reading and evidence-base log that summarises the theoretical learning that has been achieved whilst undertaking an activity. It needs to be stressed that the form of evidence selected when negotiating the learning contract should demonstrate accomplishment of the learning objective being pursued. If the learning contract is being undertaken as part of a formal education programme, the criteria for judging achievement are likely to be predetermined; however, if this is not the case, the final task in developing a learning contract involves determining the criteria and the means for validating and judging the evidence.

Learning contracts are inherently flexible, but perhaps because of the use of the word 'contract', with its legalistic tone, learners can get the idea that they may not change their learning contract once it has been negotiated. Renegotiations of learning contracts can occur at any time up until the end of the learning experience if plans or ideas change.

- Learning contracts have a number of practical benefits.
- Learners are more involved in their own learning.
- Learning contracts help learners make use of a wide variety of resources for learning, such as peers, others in the institution and community, and field experiences.
- Learners' skills of self-directed learning are sharpened, enhancing their ability to learn from experience and from their environment for the rest of their lives.
- Learning contracts provide more functional and validated evidence of the achievement learning outcomes.
- In the learning process, the conventional mentor/supervisor-imposed discipline is replaced by self-discipline.
- Learning contracts provide a way for the learner to obtain continual feedback about progress being made toward accomplishing learning goals.
- Learning contracts are more cost-effective than traditional mentor-directed learning, in that the learner is less dependent on exclusive use of the resources of mentors/supervisors and takes some of the responsibility for directing the learning off the mentors'/supervisors' shoulders (adapted from Knowles, 1986, p. 46).

However, learning contracts have some limitations: the mentor/supervisor can encounter difficulties when taking on a more facilitative role, and it can be difficult for a learner who is very new to clinical practice to contribute towards identifying their learning needs.

Key points | Top tips

Contract learning involves an agreement between at least two parties about:

- the content of the learning
- how it will be learnt
- the criteria for determining that learning has been achieved
- a diagnosis of learning needs, learning resources and strategies required
- the evidence to prove learning and a date for review of this

When implementing learning activities and evaluating learning, it may be necessary to refine the learning contract in the light of progress.

RRRRRRapid recap

Check your progress so far by working through each of the following questions.

1 Identify a minimum of four factors that are likely to affect an individual's learning?

2 What is a reason for finding out someone's learning style? Give the names of two models that could be used to do this.

3 What are the characteristics of information that can be used to help in the successful development of a learning objective?

4 What are the core dimensions of the NHS KSF and the role and responsibilities of an appraisee?

5 Identify the five key components of a learning contract or a personal development plan.

If you have difficulty with one of these questions, read through the section again to refresh your understanding before moving on.

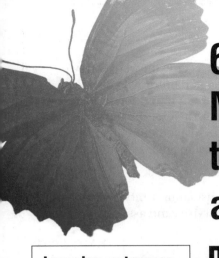

6
Mentorship, practice teaching, preceptorship and clinical supervision

Learning outcomes

By the end of this chapter you should be able to:

★ Define the main facilitator roles that support learners within practice

★ Appreciate the importance of mentorship, practice teaching, preceptorship and clinical supervision

★ Explore methods of enhancing clinical skills development and assessment

★ Value interpersonal communication and relationship building in allowing the effective giving and receiving of feedback.

🔑 Keywords

Preceptorship

involves a supportive one-to-one teaching and learning relationship between an experienced and competent role model and a newly qualified practitioner; it is for a specified time period and is to help the practitioner to adjust to their new professional role

Introduction

The relationship between the student health care practitioner and the practitioner responsible for their practice-based learning is often one of novice to expert and can be called different things depending on the professional group. For instance, nurses call this a mentorship relationship, whereas occupational therapists would term it clinical supervision. The transition from novice learner through to advanced beginner (Benner, 1984) and onwards sees the learner becoming more actively involved in setting the agenda. Although, within this chapter, I have looked at supporting practice-based learning for students under the heading 'mentorship', the content applies across professions and encompasses practice teacher working. An important stage in learning through practice occurs at the point of practitioner qualification and is termed the **preceptorship** period; this is when the newly qualified practitioner will require aid in making the transition from student to competent practitioner. As professionals settle into their qualified practice, many professions require continued formal clinical supervision, and this is looked at later in the chapter.

Although mentorship, preceptorship and clinical supervision are given separate sections within this chapter, the content relating to particular skills is relevant to all these facilitation roles. Giving and receiving feedback (included within the mentorship section), role-modelling (included within the preceptorship section), and challenging another's practice (which is incorporated in the clinical supervision section), are equally applicable to mentorship, preceptorship and clinical supervision.

Mentorship

Mentors are influential in shaping a learner's practice and therefore influence 'practice wisdom' for many years (Price, 2004). The classic concept of a mentor, used in other contexts, refers to a trusted counsellor who maintains this relationship over a period of time, and mentor relationships were originally viewed as growing between two individuals over two to 15 years. In contrast, a mentor who oversees practice learning in one placement for a student practitioner does so usually for no more than 10–12 weeks. Nevertheless, the term 'mentor' is used within nursing and midwifery for the placement clinical supervisor, whereas other health care professions more commonly use the term 'clinical supervisor'.

> A mentor is a nurse, midwife or specialist community health nurse who facilitates learning and supervises and assesses students in a practice setting.
>
> (NMC, 2005)

Practice achievement during professional courses is valued and its importance is reflected in nursing and midwifery by the 50% contribution that it makes to the achievement of a professional qualification (Andrews and Roberts, 2003). For this to be possible, sufficient appropriately experienced staff are required, and these staff need to be consistently available to support the learner in their practice placement (NMC, 2005). To undertake the mentorship role, the mentor has to be able to offer teaching, assessing, supervision, support, guidance and empathy, so that optimum learning can be achieved within the clinical placement (NMC, 2004a). Consistent engagement between student and mentor appears to have a direct impact on the learning activities accessed (Lloyd Jones *et al.*, 2001), and the mentor helps the student to understand the specific context (Field, 2004).

The quality of the student–mentor relationship has a direct influence on the development of the novice practitioner, and this is likely ultimately to influence patient care. Some practitioners seem inherently to possess the skills and qualities for mentorship, whereas others need to work on some areas: for example, a key skill is the ability to negotiate learning, and a mentor may need to work on the ability to challenge the learner's goals for their practice.

Reflective activity

- What does the term 'mentor' mean to you personally?
- What qualities and skills do you think an effective mentor should have?
- Does a mentor benefit in any way from taking on this role?
- As a student, what would you like your mentor to do?

The key components of the role of the mentor are identified here. Are these in line with what you thought during the last reflective activity?

Role of the mentor

- Identifying the needs of the learner
- Advising learners on the type of support available
- Providing guidance about facilities and learning resources in the organisation
- Following up comments from other staff about students who are performing poorly or whose conduct is unacceptable
- Referring students with particular problems to the appropriate agencies
- Carrying out assessment of learning
- Completing the practice of assessment recording on completion of the placement

Mentorship of students is often viewed as an integral part of the qualified health care practitioner's role. Some professions require additional education before the practitioner can formally take on this role: for example, Preparation for Mentorship programmes of study. Others, however, may deem that sufficient knowledge of the role can be imparted over a study day. In either case, mentors should develop a good understanding of the principles covered within the module through which the learner is progressing during their clinical placement. They need to be knowledgeable about the learning outcomes, desired competencies and the forms of evidence which can be used to show achievement of these.

Preparation for Mentorship and Practice Teaching has learning outcomes identified specifically under the following headings (NMC, 2006):

1 Establishing effective working relationships.
2 Facilitation of learning.
3 Assessment and accountability.
4 Evaluation of learning.
5 Creating an environment for learning.
6 Context of practice.
7 Evidence-based practice.
8 Leadership.

The mentorship preparation programme is delivered at a minimum academic level 2, through a minimum of 10 days' learning and is normally completed within three months (NMC, 2006). The mentor is required to have studied at the same or higher level than the student to ensure that the mentor's knowledge and skills are at a level where the complexity of practice assessment for the individual student is handled effectively (NMC, 2006). A mentor should attend curriculum development meetings, if possible, as well as educational updates (at least yearly) and link meetings as appropriate to their practice setting. The guidance from the NMC also indicates that only experienced, designated mentors and practice teachers should 'sign-off' proficiency at the end of a professional programme during the final placement period (NMC, 2006). The ability to 'sign-off' students is likely to be reviewed every three years. To help in this process, the NMC (2006) advises the use of a 'student passport' which acts as an ongoing record of achievement that is passed from one placement to another.

Placement providers are responsible for ensuring that an up-to-date, local register of current mentors and practice teachers is kept. This requires the placement provider to review the effectiveness of the mentor or practice teacher, for example, the frequency with which they take on this role and the CPD that they have undertaken. Usually, mentors should assess no more than three students at one time, and practice teachers should only have one student at a time. The NMC requires students studying for Specialist Community Public Health Nursing Advanced Practitioner or Specialist Practice qualifications to be assessed by a practice teacher (NMC, 2006).

Mentors and practice teachers must:

- be on the same part or sub-part of the register
- have undertaken CPD activities as appropriate to the role (mentorship preparation or a practice teacher qualification that is around 6 months long and has at least 30 days' protected learning time)
- hold professional qualifications equal to, or at a higher level than, those they are assessing
- be prepared to assess and support learners, including interprofessional learning.

A clinical team that views student learning as a priority may chose to identify one staff member who takes the lead in working with the educational institute and its staff. This role has sometimes been called an 'educational link'; the chosen person is also likely to be a 'sign-off' mentor or a practice teacher. This link role should improve communication between the higher education institute and the clinical team, and will help co-ordination and information sharing.

One way of assessing the potential of an individual to be a mentor/clinical supervisor/practice teacher would be to self-assess their skills and qualities using the range of 'ideal' types identified through research (Darling, 1984). The 'functions' model of mentorship, developed by Darling (1984), found 14 main dimensions:

- a **model** the student can value and admire and may wish to emulate
- a **visioner** who is enthusiastic about opportunities or possibilities and inspires interest
- an **energiser** who makes the profession fascinating and is enthusiastic and dynamic
- an **investor** who spends a lot of time with the learner, spots potential and capabilities and can hand over responsibility
- a **supporter** who is willing to listen, is warm and caring and is available in times of need
- a **standard-pusher** who is very clear about what level of performance is required and prompts the learner to achieve it

- a **teacher-coach** who can instruct about setting priorities, help to develop interpersonal skills, give guidance on patient problems and encourage learning from experience
- a **feedback giver** who can offer both positive and negative feedback and help the student to examine the things that go wrong
- an **eye opener** who inspires interest in research and is able to facilitate understanding of wider issues, such as Trust politics and departmental issues
- a **door opener** who includes the student in discussions and offers the student opportunities to be involved in new areas of practice
- an **idea bouncer** who not only discusses issues, problems and goals, but also allows the learner to present and argue ideas
- a **problem solver** who helps the student to figure out and try out new ideas and can analyse strengths and create ways to use them for the benefit of the profession or the job
- a **career counsellor** who gives guidance and support in career planning
- a **challenger** who questions opinions and beliefs and forces the student to examine decisions (adapted from Darling, 1984).

Over to you

Assess yourself in terms of these characteristics:

Table 6.1 Characteristics of a mentor (adapted from Darling, 1984)

Characteristic	This is a particular strength of mine	I can offer this	This is not a particular strength	I don't want this role
Model				
Visioner				
Energiser				
Investor				
Supporter				
Standard-pusher				
Teacher-coach				
Feedback giver				
Eye opener				
Door opener				
Idea bouncer				
Problem solver				
Career counsellor				
Challenger				

Review the boxes you have ticked and think about what areas you need to work on to improve your future mentorship/supervisory working.

The 'functions' approach can be helpful when thinking about mentorship, but it is perhaps easier to consider the key qualities and skills of a 'good' mentor.

Reflective activity

Recall a mentor or senior practitioner whom you identified in the past as a role model for your working in practice. What made this person a positive or inspiring influence?

When I asked a group of student nurses on placement in one NHS Trust, these were the factors that they suggested were displayed by 'good' mentors'.

Qualities of a 'good' mentor/clinical supervisor

- Prepared to allocate time and energy to this role
- Well-trained and supported themselves
- Has a good sense of humour and is patient, not expecting all students at the same stage in training to be the same in their clinical achievements
- Up to date with recent initiatives and prepared to be flexible and innovative
- Competent in the core skills of coaching, counselling, facilitating, giving feedback and networking
- Interested and willing to help others
- Willing to learn and can see the potential benefits of taking on the role
- Can record progress and identify the level of learning
- Able to help learners who have problems/difficulties
- Able to act as a role model

The mentor that you thought about in the last reflective activity may well have been an excellent clinical practitioner, but there is a risk that a role model may be chosen by novice practitioners without questioning their standards of practice (Andrews and Roberts, 2003). Clinical expertise is not necessarily synonymous with mentorship expertise, as the qualities and skills required are subtly different. In addition, workload pressures within senior clinical roles may adversely affect the delivery of the mentorship role. Finding dedicated time to offer learners can be a great challenge: often, mentorship is relegated to taking place 'after the work has been done'. It is crucial that the individual desires to take on the mentorship role. Doing so because there is the expectation that they should, owing to its inclusion in a job description, or in order to gain promotion is a poor basis for enthusiastic and committed learner support (Andrews and Chilton, 2000).

The NMC (2006) advises that mentors spend at least 40% of student's placement learning time (nominally 15 working hours in a full week) with their mentee. Mentors can be aware that they have not given sufficient time to their mentorship role – in one survey, only 16% of students perceived that they had received adequate contact with their mentors (Alderman, 1998) – and this may contribute to a reduction in their ability to fail students (Duffy, 2004). When the staff roster or work plan is being devised, mentor/clinical supervisor allocation should be taken into account (Price, 2004). Even when this proves difficult, some mentors are able to support learners within the limited time available because they plan learning activities, work alongside the learners when possible, and delegate mentee support through giving their colleagues associate mentor roles. It is, therefore, important to look to the wider clinical team within the mentor's health care setting as partners in supporting student learning.

Nurses are more likely to take on a clinical facilitation role if they have undertaken further studies themselves, balancing a sense of responsibility for 'good' nursing care with developing the learning culture. Mentors have shared their responsibility for learning with other qualified staff, making the 'space' for learning, and asking for confirmation of their student's learning progression (Ohrling and Hallberg, 2001a).

The quality of the mentor–student relationship influences student progress; as students learn from their mentors, they move towards practising independently under indirect supervision (Spouse, 2003). Spouse (2003) suggests that 'good' mentorship comprises four characteristics:

- befriending
- planning
- confederacy (acting as an ally)
- coaching.

A caring and trusting relationship between a mentor and student produces the most effective learning in clinical practice, and a student who is not actively 'befriended' can feel isolated and undirected (Spouse, 2003). The characteristics Spouse (2003) identifies are displayed through:

- planning prior to the expected start date of the mentee
- welcoming the mentee in a warm manner and developing rapport
- planning their time and rosters to ensure consistency of mentorship

- explaining their actions and the rationale underpinning these
- directly supporting the student when they undertake a care practice for the first time.

Mentors vary in their approach to their mentorship role, with the outcome that students receive mixed experiences ranging from highly motivated through to disinterested (Pearcey and Elliot, 2004). Failure to live up to students' expectations of mentors can be the greatest cause of disappointment in clinical practice learning for students (Pearcey and Elliot, 2004). Mentors may meet learners who appreciate the need for mentorship in a general sense, but who are not really sure of their real value. This can be helped not only by negotiating and facilitating learning but also by agreeing the 'ground rules' of the mentor–mentee relationship.

There can be negative consequences to mentoring, and it has been suggested that there is a fine line between mentor and tormentor (Feldman, 1999). There are potential pitfalls if either party enters the relationship with unrealistic expectations of time commitment or objective benefits. There can be toxic mentors, toxic protégés, and toxic environments (Feldman, 1999), and any one of these three elements can adversely affect the balance within the mentoring relationship. A mentor–mentee relationship may be dysfunctional if the needs of either party are frustrated by the relationship, if the cost of the relationship outweighs its benefit, or if specific behaviours of one sabotage the working of the other.

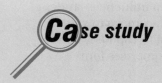

Case study

Mentorship

Julie was struggling to encourage her mentee Sandra to become interested in learning more about the drugs used within the cardiac care ward. However, Sandra seemed to feel that Julie was testing her knowledge base, and said, 'We haven't learnt about this at college yet.' Julie decided to start simply, by using examples from everyday practice on the ward. She was arranging the discharge of a patient that day, and the patient was going home on the latest ACE inhibitor*. Julie explained that she would need to discuss how the drug works, the possible problems and side effects with the patient. She asked Sandra to think about what she could do to prepare herself to help with this information giving prior to discharge. Sandra was encouraged to look up drugs from this group, e.g. Captopril, in the British National Formulary. Julie and Sandra discussed what other options there would be for finding out the information required, such as pharmacist, doctor, and other sources of drug information. Using this 'real' situation reinforced the understanding that, to work effectively in practice, a medication knowledge base is required and allowed the mentee to appreciate the need for lifelong learning regarding medication management.

What other approaches could a mentor take to a mentee who appears uninterested in furthering their learning on an aspect of practice?

*An ACE inhibitor is an angiotensin-converting enzyme inhibitor that reduces peripheral vascular resistance via blockage of the angiotensin-converting enzyme. This action reduces the myocardial oxygen consumption, thereby improving cardiac output and moderating left ventricular and vascular hypertrophy.

Assessment

The learning activities created through this patient's care could contribute towards evidence gathering for assessment of the mentee's practice during the placement. Most health care courses are now continuously assessed in practice throughout each placement. Practice assessment of clinical competence is extremely important, but confusion can be created by the multiplicity of terms used within practice-based assessment, such as competencies, learning outcomes and capability. According to McMullan *et al.* (2003) competence and competences are job related and demonstrated through performance, whereas competency and competencies are person orientated and encompass individual characteristics and qualities. If practitioners base their assessment of practice on overall competency rather than reviewing specific competences, their judgement is more likely to be subjective and difficult to demonstrate.

The practice assessment tools supplied by higher education institutes can make it difficult for mentors to recognise the essential elements of practice when assessing, but familiarity with the assessment tool makes this less problematic. Mentors and clinical educators/lecturers need to work together in the development and use of practice assessment tools to increase the likelihood of as objective a judgement as possible. In order to adequately gauge the student's knowledge, skills and attitudes, the assessment process and methodology need to be clear and understood by the mentor.

A new mentor may be anxious because they do not want to get their assessment wrong and jeopardise an individual's professional career, so they may give the student the 'benefit of the doubt' when their practice work appears to be a borderline pass/fail. It has been found that mentors who lack mentorship experience or confidence are reluctant to give a student a fail grade (Duffy, 2004).

Giving feedback

When a student is likeable and motivated but a poor achiever, it can be difficult to focus on negative aspects of their practice; but this is required if they are to progress. Not only should mentors be equipped with the ability to undertake assessment, they also need to feel comfortable with giving negative feedback. Students should also learn to take feedback constructively.

Reflective activity

Think about two occasions when you have been given negative feedback.

- The first one should be when you received negative feedback in a destructive manner. What did the person say to you? How did you feel as a result? What impact did the feedback have on your behaviour?

- Then think about a time when you received negative feedback in a more constructive manner. What did the person say to you? How did you feel as a result? What impact did the feedback have on your behaviour?

- What does this suggest to you about giving feedback to students on their practice working?

Giving students feedback means letting them know how they are performing, in a timely and ongoing way. Feedback may be formal or informal. Formal feedback is planned as part of the assessment and occurs episodically, usually covering the specific learning outcomes to be achieved. Informal feedback should be given on a daily basis in relation to specific events related to patient care. Giving negative feedback can be hard to do, but a positive critique starts when the student is asked to speak first. It is important that you own your feedback by saying 'I think' or similar. It is good to remember that criticism only improves performance when:

- it is timely and constructive
- it is given in an appropriate setting
- it is given with genuine liking for the person
- you have sought the other person's explanation
- it is related to specific instances
- it focuses on the behaviours rather than the person
- you describe the behaviour rather than judge it
- you look beneath the surface
- you look for alternative ways forward
- you allow opportunity for reflection.

Learners require constructive and informative feedback as soon as possible after the practice event if the feedback is to be meaningful, and they need to be given the opportunity to develop self-assessment and reflective skills.

> ### Over to you
>
> Read the following excerpt from a mentor–mentee midway review meeting. If you were advising the student or the practitioner what would you suggest to help improve the giving and receiving of feedback in this situation?
>
> Mentor: I wanted to mention today, because I have been thinking for a while, that your communicating with patients is not as good as it could be.
>
> Mentee: What's the matter with it?
>
> Mentor: Well (pause), sometimes you're a bit short in your communication style. You say what you need to get across to patients but you aren't very chatty or conversational.
>
> Mentee: It's really busy on here and I've been working really hard. So there hasn't been time to chat.
>
> Mentor: I know it is busy, but Angela – the other student in your group – manages to chat whilst she is delivering her care.
>
> Mentee: Angela was a nursing assistant before she came on the course, so she's more used to working on a ward.

For feedback to be effective a mentor needs to be plain speaking and specific about the action or behaviour that is being referred to. Thus, a descriptive and detailed example can be helpful. The focus should be on the actions, not the individual. There should be a balance, praising good work as well as pointing out areas that require improvement, as feedback given in this way is more likely be accepted. So in the 'Over to you' excerpt, acknowledging the hard work of the student would have been appropriate. Offering constructive suggestions of ways to improve the situation is also helpful.

Key points / Top tips

- Let the student/learner speak first
- Begin with good points
- Be specific rather than general (limit what you cover)
- Plan a solution for each problem
- Show interest, respect and involvement
- Be constructive (describe the problem that exists)
- Deal with one point at a time (give the learner time to think)
- Offer a critique of the act rather than the individual
- Do not hyperbolise (try not to use terms such as 'never', 'always')
- Do not joke
- Do not compare
- Take account of the receiver's needs
- Check that the receiver has understood
- Be productive (end on a positive note)

Receiving negative feedback

In the first moments when the student realises that they are receiving criticism, they are likely to react as anyone would: their heart beats faster and their skin temperature goes down because they feel under attack, and their first instincts are to focus on that feeling, making it more intense, which can lead to feeling like withdrawing or retaliating. On receiving negative feedback, the recipient's first instincts are to look for ways in which they themselves are right, and the momentum of defensive emotions builds fast as they focus mentally on the 'right' things that they are doing. In contrast, there is a tendency to obsess about the thoughtless, and 'wrong' things that the other person, the mentor, does. This can lead to a rigid, defensive and non-listening stance. So it is helpful if the student, when receiving negative feedback, tries to think about the good points of the mentor. They are then more likely to be generous and react calmly towards the mentor, which increases the possibility that the meeting will also look at the areas of 'good' practice in a balanced way.

Steps in responding to negative feedback

Step one: Acknowledge

- Acknowledge that you heard the mentor: for example, nod your head and pause, allowing you time to think about this and to cool down. Do not disagree or counter-attack, instead make a comment such as 'I understand you have a concern. . .'

Step two: Ask for more

- Ask for more information so that the focus is on the issue, not the feelings or personalities. Focus – mentally and/or verbally – on the aspects of the mentor that you respect.

Step three: Add your own

- If you believe the comments are accurate, acknowledge this and add your own. Then say what you plan to do differently to respond to the negative feedback; the mentor is then likely to add their actions to help towards improved practice. If you disagree with the feedback comments, ask for permission to give your reasons why, and then a constructive discussion regarding this issue can occur.

In some situations, students can feel that feedback is not very forthcoming, and if this is the case they should request it. However, when seeking feedback you need to be aware that you might hear criticism as well as praise. Try to divorce the content of the feedback from the giver and recognise that it has the potential to transform your personal and professional development.

In some cases, it is necessary for a mentor to refer or fail a student because they do not meet the necessary competencies. When this does happen, the mentor should identify this issue as early as possible to the student; it is also important that the mentor contacts the higher education institute link or contact individual. This means that support is mobilised for both the student and the mentor. The action plan that is then devised is understood by all involved, and there may be an opportunity for another assessor to add their assessment to the mentor's. Records must be kept of all discussions, action plans and any observations of practice undertaken during this period of support for a potentially failing student.

More rarely, a mentor may meet a situation where a student is unsafe in practice. This should be discussed straight away with the senior clinical lead in the practice area and the educational link from the higher education institute. It is crucial that the mentor records their reasons for deeming the student to be unsafe to continue their placement learning. This can include a written report in the practice assessment document and additionally an incident report if appropriate.

Preceptorship

A preceptor is a person who teaches, counsels, inspires, serves as a role model, and supports the growth and development of an individual (novice practitioner) for a fixed and limited amount of time with the specific purpose of assisting them into their new role. The term was first used within nursing in America in the 1970s to identify an experienced qualified nurse who, working in partnership with a newly qualified member of the nursing profession, assists the latter to adapt to their new role in a fixed period post-qualification (Morton-Cooper and Palmer, 1993). The preceptorship period within nursing is usually around 4–6 months.

Being a preceptor can be fulfilling and rewarding. The main difference between being a mentor and a preceptor is that the latter is facilitating a peer, requiring an 'enabling' relationship. Morton-Cooper and Palmer (1993) suggest that an enabler is:

- **comfortable** with themselves and their abilities
- **accessible** and able to create mutual respect
- **responsive** to others needs
- **easy to trust**.

The preceptor's knowledge of the organisation, team and clinical practice is seen as invaluable to the newly qualified practitioner, although the preceptee, as a registered practitioner, remains accountable for their actions. Preceptorship of an individual is primarily concerned with easing the transition from learner to practitioner, thereby limiting the damage of 'reality shock' (Kramer 1974), which was discussed in Chapter 3. 'Reality shock' occurs when the practitioner realises the enormity of staying within one clinical setting and taking on the responsibilities of a qualified practitioner. Through the preceptor's facilitation, supervision and acting as a role model, the newly qualified practitioner is able to achieve an effective transition from being a student.

Evidence base

Read: Tryssenar, J. and Perkins, J. (2001) From student to therapist: exploring the first year of practice. *American Journal of Occupational Therapy*, **55**(1), 19–27.
   Six students kept reflective journals over the first year of their qualified practice. From analysis of these qualitative data, four stages were identified: transition, euphoria and angst, reality of practice, and adaptation.

Recognising the stages of development within the first year of qualified practice can help those who are supporting practitioners. As well as enhancing the clinical performance and skills development of a new practitioner, the preceptorship period should help in the socialising of new team members into a practice community. It is argued that offering a formal, supportive preceptorship relationship increases staff retention, reduces stress and helps to bridge the period between the students' receiving mentorship and their progressing towards clinical supervision (Myrick and Yonge, 2001).

There can be great variations between different preceptors, preceptees, clinical settings and professional groups in their understanding and implementation of preceptorship. Although there is structured entry to many health care professions following initial qualification, the professions may well not define this as preceptorship, terming it an extension of clinical supervision.

If the needs of the preceptor, preceptee and organisation are to be met (see Figure 6.1), it is helpful if this is approached in a structured way.

The needs of a newly qualified practitioner are usually broadly based around:

- reviewing what they have achieved to date
- understanding what is expected of them
- adapting to their new role and developing new clinical skills
- continuing to learn and develop in their clinical practice
- performing effectively in their patient care
- feeling valued as part of a team.

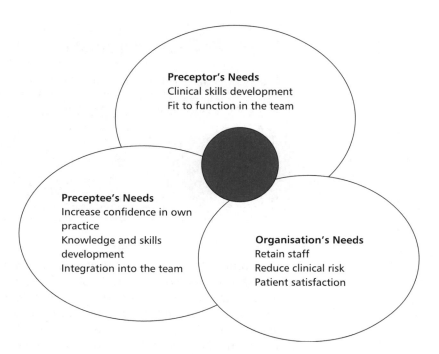

Figure 6.1 Needs to be addressed within a preceptorship learning contract

Staff in the clinical setting need to be involved in the development of a structured programme of preceptorship, including planning the preceptorship programme, involvement in education and awareness sessions and evaluating the preceptorship programme. The aim should be that all those involved identify the benefits of a structured approach and that these benefits are realised.

Key areas to formalise for preceptorship in a clinical setting

- The role of the preceptor, the relationship of the preceptor and preceptee within a preceptorship programme
- Who requires preceptorship – newly qualified staff, those returning from breaks in service and those returning after working for a significant time in a very different speciality
- The format for guidelines/documentation of the preceptorship period
- Practical issues, training and support resources available
- Linkage to current arrangements – informal structures for support

> ### ᵉˡᵗᵉᴙ*Reflective activity*
>
> Have you got what it takes to be a preceptor? Look at the attributes identified below and reflect on those you currently possess, those you would like to work on and add any others that you think are also important.
>
> | | | |
> |---|---|---|
> | advocate | role model | aware of limitations |
> | patient | flexible | organised |
> | sense of humour | knowledgeable | non-threatening |
> | enthusiasm | open to debate | effective communicator |
> | respected by peers | confident | |

When reflecting on some of the attributes of a preceptor it becomes clear that the 'toxic' preceptor would hold very different attributes, such as threatening behaviours, undermining confidence, being a poor practice model and lacking in rapport. One of the attributes you reflected on in the last activity was the preceptor as role model. Role modelling involves studying the behavioural patterns of sound professional practitioners, and it could be argued that those selected to be preceptors should be people who, the clinical team believe, meet this criteria.

> ### ᵉˡᵗᵉᴙ*Reflective activity*
>
> Reflect on your answers to the following questions.
> 1   What are the behavioural patterns of successful practitioners in the area in which you work?
> 2   How do they achieve their client-care results?
> 3   What do they do that is more successful than other practitioners?
> 4   What are the skills and qualities that make the difference?
> 5   Are these practitioners best placed to be preceptors?

Working with a role model does not mean simply replicating what they do: it involves explaining why and how one can achieve similar outcomes and requires 'thinking', as well as 'doing' in a similar way to a practitioner who is at the peak of their practice. There are three aspects to the modelling process. For instance, if a new practitioner wishes to improve their assessment skills, they will initially watch the preceptor whilst they assess a patient. During this observation, the preceptee imagines themselves doing this assessment, focusing on behaviours (what is done), internal thinking (how they do it) and the supporting assumptions, beliefs and knowledge (why they do it in that way). The 'what' is understood by direct observation, but the preceptee will only understand the 'how' and 'why' by asking questions. Having the opportunity to work alongside a 'role model' can help to increase clinical performance; however, each person brings their own unique resources and personality to a situation so this is only one strategy to help the novice practitioner.

As the preceptee is a qualified practitioner, it is important to acknowledge their individual accountability and that the preceptee must play an active part in their personal development. Preceptor qualities and skills identified as essential are leadership and communication skills, decision-making ability and an interest in professional growth. A preceptor should be willing to teach and have flexibility in providing an individualised learning experience. Support and advice should be available to preceptors to help them develop in their crucial role, and clinical supervision is an ideal forum for this. Like the mentor, the preceptor has two potentially conflicting roles – confidante and assessor – and this difficulty is further compounded by peer-evaluating another health care professional's work. Unfortunately the preceptorship period can sometimes be poorly structured; Gerrish (2000) found that some new practitioners were left to cope with little formal support.

Agreeing a set of ground rules for the preceptorship period can help 'set the scene' for an appropriate relationship, where each role and the expectations of this role are made clear. This involves setting up an individual learning contract and objectives based on the job description, competences and the knowledge and skills profile for the position. The preceptorship documentation should provide the basis for an initial Individual Performance Review (IPR) or appraisal process and the development of a further personal development plan. For further detail on how to get the most out of learning contracts, refer to Chapter 5.

During the first week of the preceptorship period, the preceptor meets with the preceptee and orientates the new practitioner to the clinical team, documentation, equipment and the communication channels in use. Any health and safety issues must also be discussed early on. Subsequent meetings are likely to focus on progress towards the learning objectives set up in the learning contract and any reflections on clinical working recorded by the new practitioner in their learning diary. Reflecting on practice in a diary can allow a practitioner to keep a record of their progress during this important time of transition and to identify any issues they want to address with their preceptor; this can lead to a re-negotiation of the learning contract. In addition to one-to-one meetings with a preceptor, it can be supportive and informative if a newly qualified staff member can continue to meet with their peer group, as this adds another dimension to their support structures at this stressful, transitional time.

Top tips

Preceptorship programmes need:

- Flexibility in the programme to meet individual needs, with allowance for a variable time scale to achieve this
- Education and support for preceptors and preceptees so that each takes an active role in the process; case scenarios are useful adjuncts to this
- A framework or guidelines for the preceptorship period, based on the practitioner competences and Foundation KSF outline (fast-track incremental progression is linked to successful achievement of preceptorship)
- Development of a learning package for preceptors, including definition, aims and objectives of preceptorship (within the NHS), role and responsibilities, training to be attended
- A formal meeting and review of preceptorship learning at approximately one-month, three-month and six-month periods, with the intention that the preceptorship period will normally be completed at the final review meeting
- A registered first-level practitioner who is already a 'sign-off' mentor, with at least 12 months' post-registration experience within the clinical setting to undertake the role (NMC, 2006)
- Preceptors with a willingness to share their skills, knowledge and attitude towards their work, and the ability to give feedback/evaluations on progress

Clinical supervision

Clinical supervision is a formal process between a skilled supervisor and supervisee that enables a professional to reflect on and assume responsibility for their practice, and develop skills, knowledge and understanding of their practice whilst feeling supported. It is advocated for all clinical practitioners as it enhances consumer protection and safety of care in increasingly complex clinical situations (NHS Executive, 1995).

Where possible, a clinical supervisor should observe a supervisee working; there should also be regular meetings. These meetings can be in a small group or just between the two individuals, and the main content is a review of recent working and the formulation of an action plan for future professional learning. The participants reflect on clinical experiences together, considering alternative ways of tackling issues, and discuss what they have learnt from the clinical experiences. They then agree how this will be applied and evidenced in the work setting in the near future.

Given the broad nature of clinical supervision, there is scope for overlap and confusion with other managerial and development activities. Supervision can take place in different formats, including clinical, managerial and training supervision. Clinical supervision enables a focus on professional competencies and high standards of the delivery of care.

Managerial supervision is concerned with the monitoring of work commissioned by an organisation. Training supervision is related to the acquisition of specific skills and competences, and accountability is often linked to an educational establishment. The learning element of clinical supervision means that there is possible confusion between clinical supervision as outlined here and mentoring students. Clinical supervision is about a professional partnership, not an expert-to-novice relationship, although many of the skills and qualities required for mentorship are also required to deliver effective clinical supervision. For instance, support is offered both verbally and non-verbally (showing concern, giving praise, listening, providing space, offering guidance and advice, showing humour, and giving time).

Reflective activity

Think about the situation where the clinical supervisor is also the line manager. Do you think confidentiality may be harder to maintain, or that it would be more difficult to establish the same levels of trust and openness?

Think about the clinical supervision in your current practice setting: what anxieties or concerns do you have about this? What possible problems have you had to contend with?

Clinical supervision should not be viewed as replacing other forms of staff support such as counselling services; however, it can make a contribution to reducing the negative outcomes of professional stress (Williamson and Dodds, 1999). Clinical supervision is an important way of developing professional skills and attributes, and this professional relationship between two qualified practitioners is ideally separate from any management structure. The focus is on individual reflection on practice, understanding and interpreting accurately the care provided with the outcome being the identification of development needs. The concept of the reflective practitioner has implications for clinical supervision on two levels – the process requires reflection on real experiences from practice, and the clinical supervision process should help develop the ability to reflect critically on practice. Supervision can take place before or after an event and can be either planned or ad hoc.

Four main themes in clinical supervision

- A formal arrangement
- Interactive partnership
- Reflection on practice
- Professional and personal development

The United Kingdom Central Council for Nursing, Midwifery and Health Visiting (1996) produced a position statement on clinical supervision for nurses and health visitors and this has been endorsed by the Nursing and Midwifery Council. The six key principles of this position statement are:

1   Clinical supervision supports practice, enabling practitioners to maintain and promote standards of care.
2   Clinical supervision is a practice-focused professional relationship involving a practitioner reflecting on practice guided by a skilled supervisor.
3   Practitioners and managers should develop their own approach to clinical supervision, taking into account local circumstances. Ground rules should be agreed so that practitioners and supervisors are aware of what is involved and can trust in the confidentiality of clinical supervision.
4   Every practitioner should have access to clinical supervision, and a supervisor should supervise a realistic number of practitioners.
5   Preparation for supervisors can be delivered 'in house' or through external education programmes, but the importance of clinical supervision should be stressed in both pre- and post-registration educational programmes.
6   Evaluation and research regarding clinical supervision are needed to assess how it influences care, practice standards and the service delivered.

Although not a statutory requirement for nurses or health visitors, clinical supervision is a statutory function for midwives, as described in the Midwives Rules and Standards (NMC, 2004b). This states that clinical supervision is considered as integral to midwifery practice and that a midwifery supervisor should have no more than 15 midwives to supervise. Clinical supervision is also integral to many other health professions: for example, clinical psychologists, counsellors, occupational therapists, physiotherapists, dieticians and social workers have already developed systems of supervision.

Changes in clinical practice, organisational roles and structures, and patient expectations continue to create new challenges for health care professionals. Whilst these new challenges may in some cases offer exciting opportunities, they also place increasing demands on the practitioners who must respond. There has, therefore, been a movement in all health care professions towards clinical supervision as a tool to combat stress, maintain standards and enhance personal and professional development. There has been growing evidence of increased stress and, in some instances, **burnout**, resulting from the conflict between the care needs of clients and the demands of the organisation.

Sufferers of burnout complain of physical, emotional and mental exhaustion which lead to a sense of reduced personal achievement and a lack of concern for patients.

⊶ *Keywords*

Burnout

Burnout is different from stress, as it causes people who have previously been highly committed to their work to become disillusioned and to lose motivation and interest.

Evidence base

In a survey of 505 public and private sector employers/employees (Hudson, 2005) it was found that:

- 52% of British employees perceived that they had experienced one or more symptoms of overwork or burnout in the last 6 months.
- Over 45% of employees and employers thought the situation had worsened in the last 5 years.
- 4% of employees believed that they were burned out or near to this.
- 8% said they rarely enjoyed work and were stressed most of the time.
- Over 75% believed that burnout was most likely due to the increased pace within work environments.

Take a look at the following journal article.

Bakker, A., Le Blanc, P., Schaufeli, W. (2005) Burnout contagion among intensive care nurses. *Journal of Advanced Nursing*, **51**(3), 276–287.
Do you think this is likely to be applicable within the health care setting?

Increased demands on experienced practitioners to support learners, when combined with already extensive responsibilities, increase the possibility of burnout (Dilbert and Goldenberg 1995). Dilbert and Goldenberg (1995), who explored the role of the preceptor, suggest that factors such as lack of support from management and other staff and insufficient time to fulfil the preceptor role alongside other duties exacerbate burnout.

The pace of change has also made it increasingly difficult for individual professionals to keep up to date with new developments and the evidence about the effectiveness and appropriateness of particular interventions or therapies. The combination of these issues can raise concern in relation to standards.

There are potential benefits for a health professional receiving clinical supervision, for the clinical supervisor, the supervisee, for the organisation in which they work, and for patients and clients.

Reflective activity

To identify the potential benefits of clinical supervision, think about the learning, supportive and quality aspects of clinical supervision and then note down the benefits for each of the following:

- the individual professional receiving clinical supervision
- the clinical supervisor
- the organisation
- patients/clients/service users.

Many researchers have tried to determine the benefits in learning and support that health care professionals gain through clinical supervision. In some cases, researchers have evaluated the use of a particular clinical supervision model: in most instances, they found that supervisors and supervisees felt generally positive about the experience of supervision. When dissatisfaction with clinical supervision is expressed, it tends to relate to supervision taking time away from direct patient care, with nurses feeling guilty for leaving colleagues to work while they receive supervision. Butterworth *et al.* (1997) found that participant benefits included the availability of time to reflect on and learn from practice, the development of self-esteem, feeling supported by peers, taking responsibility for their own practice, and feeling more honest, relaxed, enthusiastic and less competitive. However, like many researchers, Butterworth *et al.* (1997) also acknowledge that it is harder to attribute improvements in patient care directly to clinical supervision.

Clinical supervisory discussions can cover a whole range of subject or topic areas, and this is likely to vary considerably between staff. There are, however, six broad areas that are often discussed:

- clinical working or a particular case – reflecting on work experiences and developing new skills

- management and organisational working – changes in work practices, managing time and workload, staff relationships

- confidence building – exploring past actions and affirming these

- professional development – career advice, locating learning experiences/opportunities

- educational support – discussing how to coach and work with others

- personal matters and interpersonal problems affecting clinical working.

Clinical supervision is equally demanding for both supervisors and supervisees, bringing to those involved additional obligations and responsibilities if a strong supervisory relationship is to be established and maintained. The early phases of the clinical supervision relationship make a significant contribution to the overall efficacy of clinical supervision. (Sloan, 2005)

The supervisory relationship

- Generosity – in time, and being prepared to give, both emotionally and intellectually
- Rewarding – offering praise and encouragement
- Openness – to feelings, as well as providing practical skills development
- Willingness to learn – from each other
- Thoughtful and thought provoking
- Humanity – treating those involved as individuals with whom it is a privilege to work
- Sensitivity – awareness of problems
- Uncompromising – bringing rigour to the process, encouraging high standards of work
- Orientation – recognising when viewpoints may conflict and when professional opinions may conflict with the needs of the patient/client
- Trust – those involved need to maintain safety

There are different styles of clinical supervision, drawing on ideas from both leadership and teamwork. One widespread approach is to describe a continuum between a highly directive, proactive style (where the supervisor takes the decisions) and a more hands-off style (where the supervisee or group takes the decisions).

Reflective activity

Are you more comfortable in a situation where a supervisor is:

- directing and taking decisions?
- co-ordinating and sharing the decisions with you?
- space giving and letting you take the decisions?

It may be that, as the practitioner becomes more experienced, the style of the clinical supervisor should move along the range of the continuum from 'directing' towards 'space giving'. There is a range of skills and qualities that a clinical supervisor may require in order to achieve successful supervision.

> ## Over to you
>
> Assess yourself against each of the skills in Table 6.2. For each give yourself a score (tick) between 1 and 5, where 1 = a skill you need to develop and 5 = a skill you feel confident in.
>
> ### Table 6.2 Skills and qualities of a clinical supervisor
>
> | Skill/Quality | 1 | 2 | 3 | 4 | 5 |
> |---|---|---|---|---|---|
> | Facilitating reflection on practice | | | | | |
> | Demonstrating effective non-verbal listening skills, e.g. eye-contact, prompts, body posture, managing the physical environment | | | | | |
> | Demonstrating effective verbal listening skills e.g. verbal prompts, open-ended questions, repeating key words, checking impressions | | | | | |
> | Giving negative feedback | | | | | |
> | Giving positive feedback | | | | | |
> | Inspiring confidence in others | | | | | |
> | Being emotionally supportive and restorative | | | | | |
> | Dealing critically with personal and professional dilemmas | | | | | |
> | Acting as a professional resource | | | | | |
> | Self-disclosing appropriately | | | | | |
> | Setting mutually agreed goals | | | | | |
> | Preventing dependency in a professional relationship | | | | | |
> | Dealing effectively with issues of unsafe/ unprofessional conduct | | | | | |
> | Demonstrating a clear understanding of ethical rights and responsibilities | | | | | |
> | Being self-critical | | | | | |
> | Able to evaluate | | | | | |
>
> (Adapted from East Somerset NHS Trust (2000) *Clinical Supervision: Theoretical and practical approaches to the supervision of clinical practice*. East Somerset NHS Trust, Yeovil, Somerset.)

Within your review of your own skills, you may have identified dealing critically with professional dilemmas and challenging another's practice as areas for further development. Some practitioners may be less open to new ideas, and you may need to challenge someone about an aspect of their practice or in relation to the clinical supervision sessions themselves. For example, a supervisor may need to challenge the supervisee over:

- problems about how the supervisee is behaving towards a patient/client
- prejudice towards a particular client group
- problems about the way they are behaving with other health care colleagues
- errors of judgement in their professional practice
- failing to work to their professional code of conduct
- arriving late or failing to make a session altogether without an appropriate reason
- behaving inappropriately during a session
- behaving antagonistically towards another member of the supervision group.

In any of these cases, it is the responsibility of a clinical supervisor to act. In many cases, it can be enough to use the approaches to giving negative feedback, discussed earlier in this chapter. This may be sufficient for the supervisee to admit to the problem and to look to find a solution; in other cases, the supervisee may have a 'block' and change may not happen. If so, you may need to challenge the supervisee, and to confront their personal and professional blocks.

There are potential risks if we ignore the need to challenge another's practice. Hoping the issue/problem will go away and doing nothing can lead to the possibility that the situation will build up into a crisis. Challenging a colleague has the potential to be either a destructive or a productive force (see Table 6.3 below). If the situation is handled appropriately and sensitively with the problem being aired openly, the supervisor and supervisee are enabled to listen to each other and to develop new solutions.

Table 6.3 Characteristics of productive and destructive challenges

Productive challenges	Destructive challenges
Focus is on interests and facts instead of needs	Needs and personalities are emphasised
Lead to a long-term change	Lead to short-term solutions for long-standing problems
Are approached in an open manner	Are about face saving and the preservation of power
Help both supervisee and supervisor to reach their objectives	Supervisee and supervisor talk past one another, so that messages are not understood correctly and neither's objectives are reached
Are built on a bedrock of a good supervisory relationship	Damage the relationship and have the habit of being repeated

The supervisee and supervisor need to be able to communicate their feelings and thoughts clearly and honestly. There has to be a willingness to listen to the other person's point of view and to take on board their thoughts and feelings. It can be helpful to allow some time after the discussion for the supervisee to accept the challenge to their practice, so that they can separate their emotions and initial feelings about the challenge from the practical aspects of the problem. If a supervisee reacts in a manner that you were not expecting, it helps to realise that we cannot always know what 'buttons' are being pressed in the other person.

You may find the following useful when challenging another's practice.

- Remember that by demonstrating a willingness to confront difficult issues in another's practice we are doing so to encourage resolution of the problem.
- Listen to the other person carefully, to their words and observe their non-verbal signals, without interruption. This shows that you value the other person's viewpoint.
- Repeat and/or summarise the other person's discussion as this demonstrates the attention you have paid, shows active listening and may allow anything that you have misunderstood to be corrected.
- Reflect back the feelings of the other person, which may show them that you care about the feelings aroused: for example, 'It sounds like you're feeling annoyed'.
- Work with the supervisee to tackle or resolve the problem, avoiding interrupting or jumping in to judge or dismiss their ideas. (Writing notes at this point may help both of you.)
- Be aware of your communication style; tone of voice (try to speak calmly and evenly), use positive body language (give eye contact, nod, and do not fold your arms); don't interrupt but allow space for exploration of the issue, and ask open questions to encourage information to surface.

Key points | **Top tips**

- Establish a safe physical, social and psychological environment
- Focus on sustaining and developing practice
- Explore and clarify thinking
- Share information, experience and skills
- Confront personal and professional blocks
- Encourage the involvement and, where appropriate, empowerment of patients, clients and relatives
- Maintain high standards of practice
- Give clear feedback
- Explore professional accountability
- Facilitate understanding of team and organisational contracts

Approaches to delivering clinical supervision

There are a number of approaches or ways to organise clinical supervision including:

- one-to-one expert supervision (own discipline)
- one-to-one expert supervision (different discipline)
- one-to-one peer supervision
- group supervision (facilitated by a supervisor)
- peer-group supervision (may or may not be facilitated by a supervisor)
- network supervision (a group of practitioners come together from a range of localities, e.g. senior nurses from Special Care Baby Units across a region)
- cascade supervision (usually based on management arrangements, e.g. Band 7 practitioners provide clinical supervision for the Band 6 practitioners and so on).

Over to you

Each of the above approaches to clinical supervision has advantages as well as possible problems. Take three of the approaches (choose the ones you see being used more commonly in your own area of practice) and, thinking about your own locality, write down the strengths and possible problems with these forms of supervision.

Strengths and potential problems of individual supervision

Individual supervision has a number of strengths but also potential problems (see Table 6.4). In clinical supervision, the 'helping professional' takes on a role of clinical supervisor and care needs to be taken that the relationship does not take the form of a client-practitioner. Discussions about client/patient working may lead to analysis of **transference and countertransference**. Transference is the experiencing of feelings, drives, attitudes and fantasies, and defences towards a person in the present which do not befit that person, but are a repetition of reactions originating in regard to significant persons (for example, mother, father, sibling) from early childhood, unconsciously displaced onto figures in the present. Understanding and responding to transference and countertransference is an important part of working relationships and can help in the identification of 'blind spots' for clinical supervisors and supervisees. These processes may also be paralleled in the supervisory relationship (Playle and Mullarkey, 1998). However, I would suggest that clinical supervisors think carefully and use these concepts cautiously if these interpretations are to be helpful in clinical supervision and goal attainment and, more importantly, ensure that this does not cause harm.

○━┓ *Keywords*

Transference
In the traditional psychoanalytical sense, transference is defined as feeling or acting towards somebody (e.g. a helping professional) in a way that relates more to another past or present relationship

Countertransference
This occurs the other way, with the helping professional relating unconsciously to the client, based on past or current relationships

Table 6.4 Strengths and potential problems of individual supervision

Strengths	Possible Problems
Time dedicated to one supervisee, so effective working can be speedily achieved	Can be difficult to address a breakdown in the relationship
Able to create clear and focused objectives for the supervisee	Supervisee and supervisor can more easily collude, and avoid challenging existing poor practice
Input from one direction (supervisor)	Can foster dependency in the supervisee
Personalised supervisory discussions	Less diverse range of ways of working/ suggestions for the supervisee
Supervisee can work at own pace	The effectiveness of the supervisor – working is less open to evaluation
Supervisory session can be contained to around an hour and is easier to arrange as only two people involved	Transference issues may hamper clinical supervision, if unresolved
Less competitive environment	Can become a comfortable chat
Development in supervision can be easily monitored and is likely to be consistent	Evaluation and feedback is only one person's perspective

Strengths and potential problems of group supervision

Faugier and Butterworth (1992) suggest that one-to-one supervision tends to be the most frequently used approach; however, group supervision can be equally valuable (see Table 6.5). The choice of approach will depend upon a number of factors, including personal choice, access to supervision, length of experience, qualifications, and the availability of supervisory groups. In the last 'Over to you' activity you probably identified that it is important that group supervision establishes effective group working, which can take longer to achieve than in a one-to-one situation. Group supervision requires facilitation skills and an appreciation of group dynamics: for instance, an understanding of the stages of group development – forming, storming, norming, performing and adjourning (Tuckman and Jensen, 1977) – see Figure 6.2 on page 110.

It is essential that there is stability in the clinical supervisory relationships in order to develop mutual trust, respect and security: qualities that are developed during long-term relationships. This can be difficult to achieve within the clinical supervision group, where turnover of membership can pose a threat to the functional dynamics of the group. Tuckman and Jensen (1977) added the final stage – adjourning – to signal that some groups do not survive long term. As members become aware of the group's demise, they may experience sadness and remorse, and sometimes find it difficult to disengage from task behaviours.

Table 6.5 Strengths and potential problems of group supervision

Strengths	Possible Problems
Emotionally supportive atmosphere from peers	Individual's needs may not be addressed – not all are suited to group work
Can encourage experimentation with care interventions	Group members may work at varying paces
Input from many directions, e.g. supervisor and other group members	Individuals may not have the time within a session to discuss their issue or can chose to 'hide' within the group
Some supervisory discussions not about individual supervisee needs	Supervisory session needs to be longer, around two hours – difficult to arrange as a group of people is involved
Learning achieved through listening, discussing others' work and reflecting on the problems they face can be valuable	The effectiveness of the supervisor – working is less open to evaluation
Cost effective in time of the supervisor and group members	Can become a competitive environment owing to group dynamics
Less likely for dependency towards the supervisor to occur	May be lack of time for group members with large caseloads
Evaluation and feedback given from a number of people	Can be used as a 'dumping ground', where issues outside of the individuals' controls are focused on
Risk taking can be higher in group setting	Can be pressure to conform e.g. 'group think', and newcomers can find it difficult to join
Issues arising from within the group can be addressed	Lessening of confidentiality can be a problem
Reduces the power of supervisor	Individual development in supervision can be more difficult to monitor

Models of clinical supervision

There are three main categories of models of clinical supervision (Faugier and Butterworth, 1992). First, there are those that describe supervision in relation to the main functions of the supervisory relationship and its constituents (Wagner, 1957; Heron, 1989); secondly, there are models that describe the main functions of the role (Proctor, 1987), and, thirdly, there are developmental models, which emphasise the process of the supervisory relationship (Stoltenberg and Delworth, 1987). What follows is a brief overview of some of the clinical supervisory models.

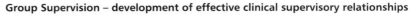

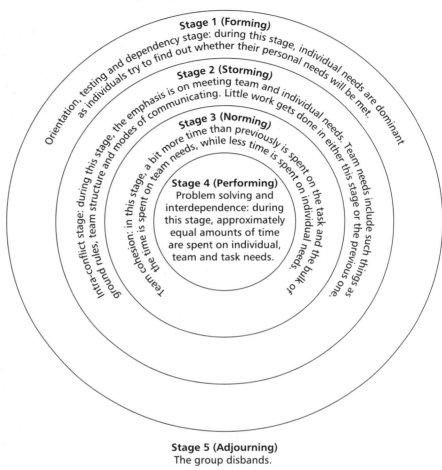

Group Supervision – development of effective clinical supervisory relationships

Stage 1 (Forming)
Orientation, testing and dependency stage: during this stage, individual needs are dominant as individuals try to find out whether their personal needs will be met.

Stage 2 (Storming)
Intra-conflict stage: during this stage, the emphasis is on meeting team and individual needs. Team needs include such things as ground rules, team structure and modes of communicating. Little work gets done in either this stage or the previous one.

Stage 3 (Norming)
Team cohesion: in this stage, a bit more time than previously is spent on the task and the bulk of the time is spent on team needs, while less time is spent on individual needs.

Stage 4 (Performing)
Problem solving and interdependence: during this stage, approximately equal amounts of time are spent on individual, team and task needs.

Stage 5 (Adjourning)
The group disbands.

Figure 6.2 *The stages of group development (after Tuckman and Jensen, 1977)*

Wagner's (1957) supervision triangle

Wagner (1957) took the view that supervisors tend to focus predominantly on one of the following three parameters.

Three modes of delivery for clinical supervision have been suggested as a way of guiding practitioners in their practice. These are:

- **Patient-centred supervision**. Supervision problems are of a technical or skills nature, and specific areas of information and evidence are sought, professional advice is given and clinical practice is monitored.

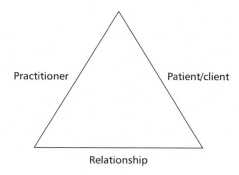

Figure 6.3 Wagner's (1957) supervision triangle

- **Clinical-centred supervision**. The focus is on unseen, unheard or unspoken components of practice through reflection on clinical events. The practitioner is encouraged to look at the dynamics involved and the factors influencing their clinical practice.
- **Process-centred supervision**. This concentrates on the processes of events between a patient, family members, colleagues, and a practitioner and their supervisor. Analogies are made between interactions that take place with the supervisor, and interactions between the patient and supervisee, sometimes termed mirroring or paralleling. This demands specific high-level supervisor skills.

Obviously, focusing on one of these at the expense of the others could limit the usefulness of the supervisory interactions.

Heron's (1989) six category intervention analysis

John Heron (1989) proposed a taxonomy for the analysis and categorisation of interventions employed during counselling, which has been used as a way to review clinical supervision interventions. The six main forms of intervention are of two types: authoritative and facilitative.

Forms of intervention (Heron, 1989)
Authoritative

- *Prescriptive* – the supervisor directs the supervisee by giving advice and direction
- *Informative* – the supervisor provides information and instructs the supervisee
- *Confrontative* – the supervisor challenges the beliefs or behaviour of the supervisee. Such confrontation does not imply aggression, rather it invites the supervisee to consider some aspect of their work or themselves that they have previously taken for granted

Facilitative

- *Cathartic* – the supervisor attempts to help the supervisee move on through the expression of thoughts or emotions previously unacknowledged or expressed
- *Catalytic* – the supervisor focuses on helping the supervisee become increasingly self-directive and reflective. They aim to 'bump up' the developmental and professional level of the supervisee
- *Supportive* – the supervisor attempts to reinforce the confidence of the supervisee through focusing on their areas of competence, and attending to what they did well

Sloan and Watson (2001) suggest that all of the intervention categories should be utilised within clinical supervision to realise the potential potency of Heron's framework.

> ## Over to you
>
> Seek the agreement of all parties involved in your supervision to record a clinical supervision interaction (make sure that this is kept confidential) then review this, filling in the following clinical supervision recording chart to show every time that the supervisor communicates. Mark which category the intervention falls within. Then discuss the review findings with all participants in the clinical supervision when you next meet.
>
> **Table 6.6 Clinical supervision recording chart (based on Heron's six categories)**
>
> | | Prescriptive | Informative | Confrontative | Cathartic | Catalytic | Supportive |
> |---|---|---|---|---|---|---|
> | 10 | | | | | | |
> | 9 | | | | | | |
> | 8 | | | | | | |
> | 7 | | | | | | |
> | 6 | | | | | | |
> | 5 | | | | | | |
> | 4 | | | | | | |
> | 3 | | | | | | |
> | 2 | | | | | | |
> | 1 | | | | | | |
>
> Discuss which interventions were used most and least frequently. Which interventions could have been used more to get the most from the clinical supervision episode?

Proctor's (1987) three function interactive model

Kadushin (1992) looked at supervision in social work and identified three main functions of supervision: administrative, educational and supportive. This way of thinking about supervision has become generally accepted, and Proctor (1987) adapted the model. The administrative function was changed to a professional or 'normative' function that includes the provision of quality control. The educative or 'formative' function was enlarged; this function enables the development of skills, understanding and abilities by reflecting on and exploring the person's work experience. The supportive or 'restorative' function provides support to enable the person to deal with what has happened and to move on.

A way of remembering this clinical supervisory model is to think of ESP.

- **E**ducational – to further develop knowledge and skills
- **S**upportive – to ensure that practitioner stability and boundaries are effective
- **P**rofessional – to maintain safe practice and satisfactory standards of care.

This framework helps in directing the balance of interactions within a clinical supervisory meeting and is also useful in evaluating the effectiveness of the relationship. However, the way that these functions are depicted tends to suggest that supervisees are in deficit, with it being the job of the clinical supervisor to help them to put things right. If this is the way that clinical supervision is viewed, the supervisor can easily slip into acting on, or upon behalf of, their supervisee.

Hawkins and Shohet (1989) have identified the primary aspects of supervision as:

- to provide a regular space for the supervisees to reflect upon the content and process of their work (Educational)
- to develop understanding and skills within the work setting (Educational)
- to receive information and another perspective concerning one's work (Educational, Supportive)
- to receive both content and process feedback (Educational, Supportive)
- to be validated and supported both as a person and as a practitioner (Supportive)
- to ensure that as a person and as a practitioner one is not left to carry unnecessarily difficult problems and projects alone (Supportive)
- to have space to explore and express personal distress, re-stimulation, transference or countertransference that may be brought up by the work (Administrative/Professional)

- to plan and utilise their personal and professional resources better (Administrative/Professional)
- to be pro-active rather than re-active (Administrative/Professional)
- to ensure quality of work (Administrative/Professional, Supportive).

Stoltenberg and Delworth's (1987) integrative development model

This model focuses on the content and process of supervision that change as the supervisee progresses in their practice.

- Stage 1 – There is reliance on the supervisor, and much of the content of supervision is based on role modelling and influencing.
- Stage 2 – This is an exploratory phase when the supervisee starts to take risks in the development of their practice and the supervisor challenges blocks and blindspots.
- Stage 3 – The supervisee takes up a position of autonomy, working on their skills and knowledge acquisition independently, and looks to the supervisor to enlarge their understanding of broader professional issues.

Although this model shows three stages that appear to progress from one to another, a practitioner might be at Stage 3 for much of their practice but also at Stage 1 for a new clinical case that they have not dealt with before.

Even though clinical supervision models vary considerably in their approach to clinical supervision, they have in common themes like supervisor–supervisee–client interaction, support, educational development, equality, shared responsibility, and the importance of a good interpersonal relationship.

Practical arrangements for clinical supervision

Clinical supervision contracts are usually recommended as this helps ensure clarity of roles and responsibilities, and is likely to formalise the need to undertake adequate preparation. Supervision contracts help to:

- prepare for a situation where supervisee and supervisor have different expectations of supervision with a subsequent reduction in the effectiveness of the supervisory relationship
- negotiate mutual expectations at the formative stages of supervision to help avoid problems later in supervision
- ensure working in supervision is structured, collaborative and begins to establish a pattern of attention in supervision to the process, content and relationship in order to be reflexive
- establish professional boundaries through making explicit the developmental, professional and legal functions of supervision
- create an underpinning foundation so that both supervisee and supervisor feel safe and supported.

Decisions to be made in agreeing the clinical supervision contract include:

- the type of supervision offered e.g. peer, one to one
- ground rules and policy regarding confidentiality
- suitability of the type of supervision to the supervisee's current needs
- the clinical supervision model and techniques that will be used
- the emphasis of the supervision, e.g. process, content and relationship
- practical considerations, e.g. meeting room, frequency, duration, note taking
- goals, aims and objectives of clinical supervision and the need to make them SMART (Specific, Measurable, Attainable, Relevant and Time limited)
- the rights and responsibilities of both the supervisee and supervisor
- how the effectiveness of supervision will be measured/evaluated
- how any problems will be handled from both the supervisee's and supervisor's perspectives
- how issues that are outside the competence of the supervisor will be handled
- how poor or incompetent practice will be addressed from both a supervisee and supervisor perspective
- the process of review and renegotiations of the supervision contract.

From the previous exploration of clinical supervision, and taking into account the need to challenge blocks in practice and to find time within a busy clinical schedule to meet, it becomes clear that it is necessary for those involved in the supervision process to agree **'ground rules'** at the start.

Ground rules for supervision commonly cover confidentiality, complying with codes of professional conduct and treating each other with respect.

⌐ Keywords

Ground rules
Ground rules are an agreed set of standards that allow meaningful dialogue to proceed with the aim of minimising conflict and increasing the effectiveness of the pair/group. To be effective, the rules must be agreed upon by everyone involved beforehand. Any deviation in practice away from the agreed ground rules should be reviewed by those involved

Over to you

If you are already involved in clinical supervision (either giving or receiving), review your ground rules and determine whether these need updating or revising in the light of what you have learnt from this chapter.

If you are not in a supervisory relationship construct at least four rules that you would like to see in a set of ground rules for your future supervision.

When, where and how long the supervisee and supervisor will meet needs to be planned and rostered into clinical working arrangements. It is common to meet from once a month to every six weeks; one-to-one supervision is likely to require at least 45 minutes to one hour; group supervision will require longer (but no more than two hours). A time needs to be identified that suits everyone; it should be when people are less likely to be called upon or interrupted. An appropriate place needs to be arranged where supervisory discussions can go ahead in confidence without risk of being disturbed or overheard. Contact details should be updated regularly in case any arrangements need modifying.

Within sessions it is vital to manage time, sticking to agreed timings for each session, monitoring how long is spent on each topic, and highlighting potential risks before they occur. Participants in the supervision session will need to agree how the agenda for the meeting is set, and what will happen if a discussion runs over time. In some cases, a supervisor may need to bring a discussion gently, but firmly, to a close. It is vital to finish sessions on time, allowing time at the end of the session to review what has happened and plan the actions to be taken prior to the next session.

Clinical supervision does not necessarily involve records; however, this can help in ensuring that the arrangements remain formal. It is perhaps wise for the supervisee to take responsibility for safe storage of these, and it should be stressed that these should not include patient/client details.

Implementing clinical supervision

An organisational and departmental culture may have a direct impact on your success as a clinical supervisor (Grant, 2000). Problematic dynamics can occur when there is a perceived lack of collaboration or involvement on the part of the manager, supervisor or supervisee; three major stakeholders in any implementation of clinical supervision.

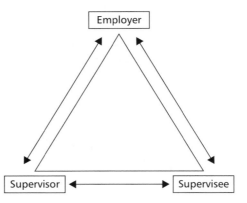

Figure 6.4 The three-cornered contract in clinical supervision (adapted from English, 1975)

In the three-cornered contract illustrated above, the desired situation exists where the contract and expectations are clear on all sides, all role definitions are clear and there are no hidden agendas.

Problematic dynamics can include the following:

- Although supervisor and supervisee feel that they are on the same wavelength, both feel distant from their employers, who do not seem interested in supporting clinical supervision.

- Employer and supervisors are clear about their goals and actions, although there is considerable distance between them and the supervisee. The supervisee may be reluctant to take up the supervision opportunity and may view the supervisors as having a management-oriented evaluative role.

- The supervisor is seen as an outsider by both the employer and supervisee, leaving the supervisor feeling both psychologically isolated and that they value clinical supervision differently from others.

Despite these potential problems in implementing clinical supervision and other clinical facilitation roles, health care professions have shown increasing interest in receiving clinical supervision and reflecting upon the nature of their own learning needs.

RRRRRRapid recap

Check your progress so far by working through each of the following questions.

1 What are the main differences between mentorship and preceptorship?

2 How should a mentor handle a situation where a student is performing poorly and is at risk of failing their practice assessment in the placement?

3 What issues need to be decided in order to formalise a preceptorship programme?

4 Define 'clinical supervision' and name two models/frameworks for clinical supervision.

5 Why are ground rules necessary within clinical supervision?

If you have difficulty with one of these questions, read through the section again to refresh your understanding before moving on.

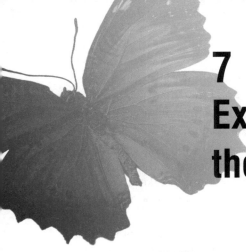

7
Experiential learning and the role of reflection

Learning outcomes

By the end of this chapter you should be able to:

★ Define the concepts of peer learning, problem-based learning and praxis

★ Utilise reflective frameworks to review practice decision-making

★ Explore team facilitation and action learning

★ Value evidence-based practice and pragmatic approaches to action-planning.

Introduction

In a single day, a health care professional has to make many rapid decisions about how to respond to unique and complex situations. Yet they often seem to practise with little in the way of conscious reasoning. So how are those decisions made? Within this chapter, we will explore some of the 'scaffolding' that can help keep decisions 'on track'.

For instance, in conditions where there is too little time and many interruptions, nurses have been found to compensate by developing a range of strategies, including minimising the time spent doing tasks, creating time and redefining the work that has to be done by prioritising and reprioritising (Bowers *et al.*, 2001). Nurses work at a fast pace and combine tasks (e.g. documenting a patient's fluid intake whilst watching the patient take their medication). They change the sequence of tasks (e.g. documenting care long after its delivery), and communicate their heavy workload to patients to reduce any possible additional requests. They 'make time' by coming in early, missing meals or doing work at home (Bowers *et al.*, 2001). The underlying pattern is one of trying to maintain continuity for patients while completing as many physical tasks as possible.

In the course of this chapter, we will explore how individuals and clinical teams can work on their conscious decision-making regarding patient care. Practice involves the gaining of new knowledge by developing and applying methods that draw from situated, individual instances of practice, with practitioners critically examining practice through systematic self-reflection, reflective discourse, and critically oriented change.

Experiential learning

As professional knowledge is functioning, specific and pragmatic and deals with determining priorities and executing actions, problem-based learning appears to be a suitable method of facilitating learning.

Problem-based learning starts with problems or situations rather than with the exposition of knowledge; it is sometimes called context-based learning or inquiry-based learning. Biggs (2003) considers problem-based learning to be a total approach to teaching that reflects the way that people learn in real life where they simply get on with solving the problems that life puts before them with whatever resources are to hand.

The eight tasks of problem-based learning (Wolff and Rideout, 2001) have been identified as:

1   Explore the problem, clarifying terms and concepts, creating hypotheses and identifying issues.
2   Identify what you already know that is pertinent.
3   Identify what you do not know.
4   Prioritise the learning needs, set goals and objectives, allocate resources.
5   Engage in a self-directed search for knowledge.
6   Share knowledge and information effectively with others.
7   Apply, use and explain the knowledge and skills.
8   Reflect on what has been learnt and the process of learning.

The 'coaching' approach to supervising learning in problem-based education encompasses goal setting, modelling, guiding, facilitating, monitoring, and providing feedback to learners to support their active and self-directed thinking and learning. Problem-based learning is different from conventional problem-solving learning, where the learners are set a problem or case after they have been taught the knowledge (Savin-Baden, 2000). Biggs (2003) suggests that it is important to align learning outcomes, teaching and learning activities, and assessment tasks in problem-based learning to encourage deep, rather than surface, approaches to learning.

Since Dewey (1938) argued that all learning can be viewed as experience, there is now growing consensus that experiences form the basis of learning. Professional learning, which integrates theory within practice in the workplace, challenges the curricular assumptions on which many health care programmes are based, meaning that experiential knowledge is professional practice (Richardson, 1999). One way of defining experiential learning was developed by Kolb (1984b, p. 38), who viewed this as 'the process whereby knowledge is created through the transformation of experience'. (Further discussion of Kolb's learning cycle is contained in Chapter 5.) Usher and Soloman (1999) view experiential learning as experience constructed in a particular way. This differentiation between everyday experience and experiential learning is not about devaluing experience but reinforces the need for intent in the process of learning within practice settings in order to build knowledge.

Reflective activity

Think about the key findings from the research study by Bowers *et al.* (2001) mentioned in the introduction to this chapter. Within this long-term nursing care facility for older people, the nurses were observed to be applying a range of strategies to 'keep up' with the physical care demands of the work setting. Have you seen this happening within clinical placements? Have you been aware of using some of these strategies yourself? What role do you think reflective processes could play in exploring the effects of these strategies?

The learning cycle starts with experience, proceeds through reflection to action, which in turn becomes concrete experience for further reflection. Experiential learning can be relatively independent of organising or mediation and takes many forms, including not only structured clinical placement experience, simulation, role-play and involvement in a change-management project but also any form of personal development. Involving others in experiential learning, for instance through action learning, allows proposed actions and their consequences to be exposed to constructive criticism.

Praxis

Praxis is a complex activity by which individuals become critically conscious human beings using a cycle of action–reflection–action that is central to learning. Characteristics of praxis include self-determination, proactive intention, creativity and conscious decision-making. Phronesis – a process of moral reasoning enacted to establish the 'good' of a particular situation and often referred to as practical wisdom – is central to the concept of praxis (Connor, 2004). Rolfe (2006) suggests that the model in which theory is viewed as informing and controlling practice should give way to a model in which theory and practice are seen as mutually enhancing, with theory being derived from practice, and in turn influencing future practice. He refers to this coming together of theory and practice as nursing praxis, and he suggests that informal theory should be unique to each individual encounter with a patient. A clinical practitioner is also, therefore, a theorist and a researcher who responds to patients by the process of reflection-in-action, drawing upon the practitioner's expertise and a repertoire of past experiences and encounters.

- Learners are actively involved in an exploration of an experience
- Experiential learning involves a cyclical sequence of learning activities
- Learners should critically and selectively reflect on their experience
- Learners should be committed to the experiential process
- There needs to be scope for the learner to explore the experience independent from the facilitator/clinical supervisor

Reflection

There is a common-sense view of reflection that sees this as a way of thinking or mental processing that is done to achieve an outcome or purpose: for example, the thoughts we might have as we drive home from work, mentally reviewing the day. However, reflective learning in professional and academic contexts is likely to involve a conscious process of critical review, clarification and actions which in some instances is transformative in revising the meanings underpinning judgements.

Dewey (1938) was one of the first theorists to define reflection; he identified it as turning over in your mind a subject and giving it serious consideration. Reflection involves the movement away from acceptance of information, which novices may do, to questioning and becoming active in critically thinking and learning. Boyd and Fales (1983, p. 100) define reflection as 'the process of internally examining and exploring an issue of concern, triggered by an experience, which creates and clarifies meaning in terms of self and which results in a changed conceptual perspective'.

Reflective practice can be summarised as having three components: experience–reflection–action, termed the ERA cycle (Jasper, 2003). These are:

1 experiences that happen to a practitioner
2 the reflective processes that allow the practitioner to learn from these experiences
3 the actions that result from the new perspectives that are achieved through reflection.

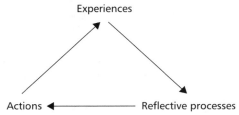

Figure 7.1 The ERA cycle of reflective practice (adapted from Jasper, 2003)

Reflective processes include an opportunity to look at the context in alternative ways allowing us to focus on different aspects of our experiences. Cowan (1998) distinguishes between analytical and evaluative reflection: the former answers the question 'How do I do it?' and the latter 'How well can I do it?' The evaluative aspect of reflection is critical in the sense of exercising discernment and making judgements. Without such critical evaluation it would be difficult to complete the reflective process and for the learning from reflection to result in action and improvement.

Scanlon and Chernomas (1997) have suggested an alternative three-stage model of reflection:

1. awareness – initiating reflection through discomfort, lack of information or seeking an explanation

2. critical analysis – taking into account current knowledge, critically examining and thinking about the event/issue

3. new perspective – outcome of analysis and new information which leads to changes and actions/outcomes.

The connection between critical thinking and reflection is evident in much of the health care and education literature.

The process of reflection is complex and involves making a judgement on experience and making assessments in the light of a standard (either personal or drawn from others' experience). What has sometimes been omitted from a discussion of the experiential learning cycle is the need for decisions to be made. When learners systematically engage in critical thinking, they tend to develop insights into their learning processes and practice.

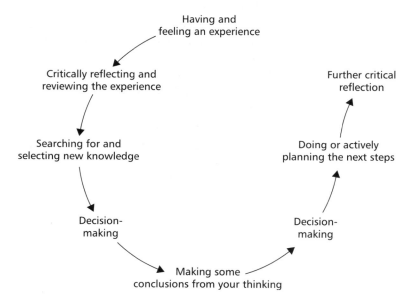

Figure 7.2 The learning cycle and decision-making (after Rogers, in Leeper, 1967)

The discussion in Chapter 5 on learning styles has made you aware of the possibility that some learners may find it difficult to think reflectively. Non-reflection is evident when a person simply mentions or describes a concept, for example, a habitual way of working, and makes no attempt to expand on this and relate it to their future working. This is termed Level 1 by Hatton and Smith (1995) who posit four levels of reflection:

1 description – pure description with no reflection

2 descriptive reflection – a description of the event; the possibility of alternative viewpoints is accepted, but mostly the reflection is from one perspective

3 dialogic reflection – able to step back from the event and actions and to explore and analyse these, recognising inconsistencies and that differing judgements and alternative explanations exist

4 critical reflection – shows an awareness of the event and actions from multiple perspectives, understanding the influence of social and political context.

The level may affect the overall outcome of reflection, as higher-level reflection should increase clarity and personally valuable learning. Hatton and Smith's (1995) level descriptors help in encouraging students or qualified professionals to deepen their reflective skills, but you need to be aware that undertaking critical reflection requires an ability to determine an endpoint so that reflection is practical and manageable.

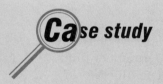
Case study

Student (community specialist practice – health visitor)

I am at the stage when I have started to take on a supervised caseload of my own. When I came out of a 'new birth' visit to an 11-day-old baby boy and his mother, my practice teacher said she felt that the mother could be at risk of developing postnatal depression – despite the fact that she had no evidence to base this on apart from her experience and intuition. I found myself thinking, is she right, and if so will I ever feel that expert and confident?

At the next follow-up visit to this first-time mum, she appeared very happy and not as though she was suffering from classic postnatal depression. My practice teacher sat patiently and listened to the client, waiting for me to take up an opportunity to ask her about her feelings. I sat anxiously, watching what was going on and trying to work out what it all meant. Eventually, I plucked up the courage to discuss how the mother was really feeling and we filled in the Edinburgh Postnatal Depression Scale questionnaire. It became clear that the mother was relieved that we had given her an opportunity to discuss how she was feeling. She had some insight into the possibility that she may be suffering from postnatal depression and she was willing to have professional help. The mother seemed fairly comfortable with the outcome of the visit, as did my practice teacher, but this left me feeling concerned as to whether I would have been able to pick this up were I to be practising on my own as a newly qualified health visitor. Will I be able to develop the same level of expertise in recognising postnatal depression?

continued

As a learning experience this was very useful. I identified a deficit in my knowledge base and my practice skills. We use the Edinburgh Postnatal Depression Scale, which was developed by Cox in the 1980s for use as a screening tool. It is a self-administered questionnaire consisting of 10 statements each with four possible responses, which are scored from 0 to 3 linked to perceived severity. A score of 12 or above is an indication of possible postnatal depression when combined with a clinical interview. This woman scored 13, and I now feel confident in using this to differentiate between feeling tired. . . tearful and suffering from postnatal depression.

What insight does this student health visitor show through this reflective account?
What level of reflection as devised by Hatton and Smith(1995) would best describe this reflective account?
What additional elements could be added to this reflection to strengthen this further?
Reference: Cox, J.L., Holden, J.M. and Sagovsky, R. (1987) Detection of postnatal depression: development of the Edinburgh Postnatal Depression Scale. *British Journal of Psychiatry*, **150**, 782–786.

Reflection often involves the highlighting of past emotional experiences. In the above case study, the student health visitor had not picked up the cues regarding possible postnatal depression but her practice teacher had, an example of the experienced practitioner knowing more than they may make explicit to a student. The expert practitioner (Schön, 1983) uses knowledge and skills influenced by attitudes to solve problems in the work place. This problem-solving process is automatic, routine and intuitive and requires little critical thinking, and has been termed reflection-in-action. Reflection-in-action is where:

- the potential range of outcomes are recognised

- the problem is reviewed and alternative hypotheses thought about

- further information is sought (either from the patient or from sources of professional knowledge, e.g. colleagues, literature).

Reflection-on-action, however, involves the situation – for example, new practice, existing practice or outmoded practice – being reviewed after the event and this leads to new learning. This retrospective process often raises questions that require further information, professional knowledge or self-inquiry. So this process adds to the development of a zone of mastery. Schön (1983) identified an interaction – in the form of **synergy** – between practical competence and professional artistry and hence learning.

Although professional training is based on a common knowledge or skill set, as soon as an individual engages in assessing and responding to specific patient needs that individual's practice becomes differentiated from that of others. Practice is prevented from becoming routine owing to the uniqueness, ambiguity and potential conflict within any clinical situation. Reflection may not be an easy process to master and can be a challenge to encourage in others. Many writers have suggested strategies

◦━ℝ Keywords

Synergy
The result of two agents, forces, people or groups coming together that leads to an enhanced outcome that is greater than the sum of each part

or frameworks for developing reflective abilities, which usually offer a series of questions or tasks to help the person advance their thinking beyond the taken for granted. This more structured approach to reflection gives time and space for thinking, what Barnett (1997) terms 'intellectual space', and also allows ownership of the learning.

Reflecting on critical incidents

Most frameworks start with selecting an experience, such as an incident from practice. When a health care professional chooses an incident to reflect on, this is usually because it is significant for some reason or has a particular meaning: perhaps it is linked to an area of practice which is an identified learning need, or it relates to a difficult clinical situation where the outcome was unexpected or unwanted. Flanagan (1954) first used the term 'critical incident': such an event may be a positive or negative experience that is suitable for description in a reasonably concise way. Unfortunately, the term 'critical incident' has sometimes been misunderstood within health care, as the word 'critical' is often used to mean 'serious'. Flanagan (1954) intended 'critical' to mean something that stands out in some way. Confusion has also crept into the discussion of reflective strategies because of the idea that all stimuli for reflection come from critical incidents that have caused us uncomfortable feelings or discomfort. This is not the case: although reflection is often stimulated by unpleasant or uncomfortable feelings, much can also be gained by examining when things go well in order to build on or replicate this situation.

The stages of reflection or critical incident analysis are listed here:
Stage 1 – selecting an experience to reflect on
Stage 2 – describing the incident
Stage 3 – analysing the experience
Stage 4 – interpreting the experience
Stage 5 – exploring alternative perspectives on the incident
Stage 6 – moving to action.

Reflective activity

Consider a recent experience in your own practice where you found yourself faced by a new problem or situation and were not sure about how to act. How did you reflect on the experience? What does this tell you about your use of reflective processes?

Recollections of an event change over time: closer to an event the focus is likely to be on the emotions that were displayed and the reactions to the situation; whereas, an individual may be able to think more broadly about the situation when time has elapsed. If a learner is being encouraged to discuss and reflect on a clinical incident, it can be helpful to keep written records as these allow the clinical supervisee and supervisor/mentor to revisit the records over time which is something that purely verbal reflection may not allow.

Having described the experience, the practitioner then starts to draw conclusions from what has been described and discussed. During this stage, they should be encouraged to develop a deeper understanding of the experience by exploring certain aspects of it in detail and coming to an explanation. Once an explanation has been ascertained, those involved in the reflective process can then go on to explore the alternatives.

Exploring the alternatives can be challenging, as to get the most from this part of the process the person is asked to move beyond how they have previously perceived the incident and look at different ways of understanding it. A mentor or clinical supervisor can help in offering a different way of viewing a situation, widening and deepening the learner's understanding. Identifying alternative perspectives helps the person who is reflecting to identify actions that they could take based on this new learning.

The mentor should try to make sure that the learner focuses on their own actions, weighing up the consequences of particular actions and recognising that these must be within their sphere of control. It can be too easy just to expect others to act for them, or for others to change themselves. The mentor may also learn from this reflective activity and decide to change their ways of dealing with something as a consequence of discussing their mentee's experience. Taking action can be viewed as the final part of the reflective process, but, as reflection is cyclic, it is likely that the health care professional will undertake further reflection about the actions taken.

Frameworks for reflection on practice

There are many frameworks that can be used to encourage reflection on practice, and learning through reflection may be more potent if there is structure to guide the act of reflection. Some models to help you engage in the process of reflection are now discussed. There is no right one; it is important that you choose and adapt the framework that feels most comfortable for you and best assists you in learning from your experiences. One well-known framework was developed by Graham Gibbs (1988); he proposed a cycle of reflection comprising six stages and a series of cue questions to guide a practitioner through each stage of the reflective process.

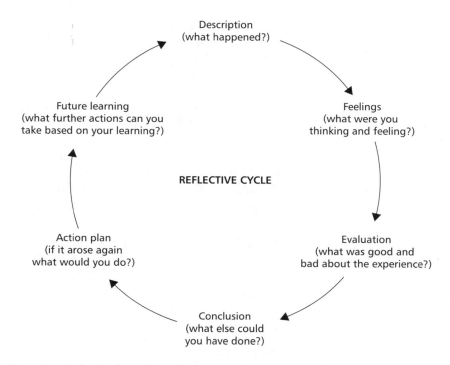

Figure 7.3 Reflective Cycle (adapted from Gibbs, 1988)

The framework devised by Palmer *et al.* (1994) also offers cues that you may find useful for structuring your reflective learning. As you will see, it is quite a simple set of questions.

Reflective framework
(adapted from Palmer, Burns and Bulman, 1994)

Choose and describe a situation you wish to reflect on. Ask yourself:

- What was my role in the situation?
- Did I feel comfortable or uncomfortable, why?
- What actions did I take?
- Who else was involved in the situation and how did they act?
- Were these actions appropriate?
- How could I have improved the situation for myself and others involved?
- What can I change in the future?
- Do I feel I have learnt anything new about myself?
- Did I expect anything different to happen? If yes, what?
- How has this situation changed my thinking?

Keywords

Epistemological
Examining the nature of knowledge and human understanding, including how knowledge is derived, determined, validated and tested

Johns' (2000) structured reflection model provides a series of cue questions based on a description of the experience, reflection, influencing factors and learning. Johns has revised his reflective framework many times, incorporating Carper's (1978) 'ways of knowing', discussed previously in Chapter 2, and this is a strength of the model, which is one of the few models of reflection to refer to the development of an **epistemological** base to reflections.

Model of reflection (Johns, 2000)

Looking in

- Find a space to focus on self.
- Pay attention to your thoughts and emotions.
- Write down those thoughts and emotions that seem significant in realising desirable work.

Looking out

- Write a description of the situation surrounding your thoughts and feelings.
- What issues seem significant?

Aesthetics

- What was I trying to achieve?
- Why did I respond as I did?
- What were the consequences of that for the patient/others/myself?
- How were others feeling?
- How did I know this?

Personal

- Why did I feel the way I did within this situation?

Ethics

- Did I act for the best? (ethical mapping)
- What factors (either embodied within me or embedded within the environment) were influencing me?

Empirics

- What knowledge did or could have informed me?

Reflexivity

- Does this situation connect with previous experiences?
- How could I handle this situation better?
- What would be the consequences of alternative actions for the patient/others/myself?
- How do I now feel about this experience?
- Can I support myself and others better as a consequence?
- How available am I to work with patients/families and staff to help them meet their needs?

Additional useful information is also supplied (in Table 7.1 below) for Johns' (2000) question, 'What internal factors were influencing me?'

Table 7.1 Internal factors

Expectations from self: – obligation/duty – conscience – beliefs/values?	Negative attitude towards the patient/family?	Expectations from others: – in what way?
Normal practice – felt I had to conform to a certain action?	What factors influenced my actions?	Loyalty to staff versus loyalty to patient/family?
Fear of sanction?	Time/priorities?	Anxious about ensuing conflict?

Reflective activity

In the previous reflective activity within this chapter, you were asked to consider a recent experience in your own practice where you found yourself faced by a new situation. Using the cue questions from Johns' framework, write down the answers that relate to this recent experience. Then compare your learning, identified through your previous reflection, to undertaking reflection using this structured approach.

Have you gained any new insights?

Reflection helps the learner who is trying to understand meaning, but some learners may have difficulty with this way of learning and may be resistant (Boud and Walker, 1998), as their peer group's cultural norms may be more 'scientific' and this approach might be thought of as 'too woolly'.

Borton's (1970) developmental framework can assist practitioners to make sense of and then respond to real clinical situations. Borton asks the person to reflect using three basic starting points to the questions. These starting points for reflection and sample cue questions are supplied on page 130.

Developmental framework (Borton, 1970)

1   WHAT? (Describe)
2   SO WHAT? (Theory and knowledge building)
3   NOW WHAT? (Action)

The 'what' cue questions could be, for example:

- What happened?
- What were you doing?
- What were others doing in this situation?
- What were you trying to achieve?
- What was good or bad about the experience?

The 'so what' cue questions could be, for example:

- So what additional information do I need to know in order to understand the situation?
- So what could I have done that was different?
- So what did I base my actions on?
- So what did those involved in this situation learn?

The 'now what' cue questions could be, for example:

- Now what should I do?
- Now what do I need to do to make things better?
- Now what might be the consequences of this action(s)?
- Now what contextual issues do I need to look at?

> ### Over to you
>
> Take a look at Jasper, M. (2003) *Foundations in Nursing and Health Care. Beginning Reflective Practice*. Nelson Thornes, Cheltenham.
> Read the section on Borton's framework and 'What? So What? Now What?' and try using the additional cue questions given in your own reflection.

Problems encountered when using reflection as the basis for learning are usually due to inexperience or misunderstanding. For example, when models of reflection are used as checklists for learners to work through in a methodical manner without any regard to their personal issues, there is a risk that reflection becomes ritualised and 'recipe following' (Boud and Walker, 1998). Facilitators of reflection need to be aware that reflection leads to serious questioning, and this means not only that it cannot be contained within a 'comfort zone' but also that it can foster a critical approach to understanding the clinical context. Reflection can also become rather intellectualised, with feelings and emotions being denied or lessened. Trusting others with our reflections inevitably involves risk, and enabling enough trust for emotional disclosure creates challenges for all involved. When facilitating reflection we may make assumptions about a particular event (Boud and Walker, 1998), and it can be taxing to respect learners and their agendas and take these as the focus rather than the agendas of the clinical placement area. Despite this, reflective processes are crucial to experiential learning and are something worth working on.

Key points **Top tips**

- Build on the way you reflect already. Try becoming more aware of how, when and why you reflect on things
- Put time aside to reflect on a regular basis, and take up opportunities to share your reflection with others, e.g. your clinical supervisor
- Try using a structured approach, e.g. a framework with cue questions, as a starting point for developing your own methods
- If you keep your own 'reflective journal or diary', read over the entries on a regular basis and look for themes
- Consider how far you are reaching any goals or taking actions you set yourself as part of reflecting
- Look for changes in yourself, your actions, attitudes, confidence and practice
- Notice and celebrate your achievements
- Be positive about the process: it takes time for progress to be made, but you will see the benefits of reflection over time

---

Action learning

Action learning involves the application of the experiential learning cycle to work activities; it is linked to action research and structured reflection and shares the same processes. Action learning aims to help individuals and teams free themselves from any oppressive structures and taken-for-granted aspects about their everyday practice (Manley *et al.*, 2005) and builds on the strengths of students and staff by using a solution-focused approach.

Action learning involves five stages:

1 Reflect on current working.

2 Develop a plan of action to improve what is already happening.

3 Implement the plan.

4 Observe the effects of the action.

5 Reflect on these effects as a basis for future action planning.

There is, therefore, a continuing cycle of improvement based on evidence, in its broadest sense, and the practicalities of the clinical setting. The starting point for a cycle of action learning might be an observation of a problem in your own clinical setting. For example, a nurse might notice that the two teams delivering care on a ward often have varying workloads, and some people within the team feel overloaded. Some reflection on this problem might lead to the analysis that responsibilities have not been divided up appropriately or that the geographical divisions of patient care within the team need to be reconsidered. An action plan might involve changing some individuals' responsibilities or a change in the patient assignment method for the two teams. The ward staff could then operate for a specified time period with the new responsibilities/patient allocations, during which time the effect on workloads, team morale and delays in getting jobs done could be monitored. At the end of the trial period, all team members could contribute through reporting back as to whether the change in practice has been beneficial. This action learning cycle could lead to a new understanding of how to share the work more effectively within the ward.

An action learning team (often termed 'set') is based on the relationships between individuals in the group and they then plan future action within the structured attention and support of the group. Put simply, action learning is about solving real problems and getting things done, and it can be a method of personal management and organisational development.

Reflective activity

What possible anxieties or concerns would you have if your clinical team decided to use action learning as a method of working on improvements in the clinical setting?

○─ㅠ *Keywords*

Empathy

The willingness to share and understand another person's feelings and thoughts, so that you can help them to solve their own problem. Cultivating empathy, the ability to appreciate and believe how it feels to be in another's shoes, leads to more trusting relationships

It is important to have **empathy** with participants in action learning sets who have a 'problem'. It is useful to cultivate an attitude that is curious and thoughtful about the way the person feels about the problem under discussion. This enables participants to be more open about their problem, and, in being so, they discover issues of which they were themselves previously unaware.

It is usually the case that each person in a set would have a slightly different reaction if they were in the same situation. For this reason, it can be unhelpful to describe 'what I would do in your situation'. One way to approach this is simply to ask 'How do you feel about. . .?' The answers are often surprising and help the participant to recognise their own feelings about an issue.

Action learning is a method that helps participants to develop by learning from each other, and it is a structured way of tackling everyday problems in a supportive yet challenging and informed way. The method requires team members to come together on a regular basis to share their problems and experiences. There are usually three stages: identifying and clarifying the problem, listing possible actions, and selecting which specific action to take. Although there may be team 'problems' to tackle, members of an action learning set retain responsibility for working on and solving their own problems.

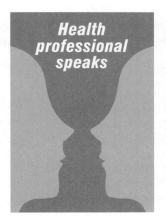

Health professional speaks

Action learning participant

This was the first time I had been involved in action learning, although I have obviously worked in many group or team situations before. I hadn't thought about how much I enjoyed it until we came to the end of the project. I reflected on why I had enjoyed this particular group work so much. Part of it was because the group members were very dedicated to the group and really easy to get along with. I now see that it was also more related to the fact that we spent quite a time early on in group-building functions, such as the development of ground rules. We also worked on maintaining the group, by keeping notes and holding people to agreed actions. I now realise there was a lot of co-ordinating, facilitating, supporting and encouraging going on. This has made me consider how I will set up future team meetings and group working.

If members of a clinical team work together as an 'action learning set', they can start to improve their performance by taking action and then reviewing their results. Sometimes, a facilitator can help others in learning about key problems within everyday experience and by reviewing progress. Whilst planning and initiating team or care delivery changes, set participants also have an opportunity to review their own development needs and try out personal changes. As a result, set participants improve their own and their organisation's performance. Action learning sets can enable participants to make commitments to action that they would not necessarily be in a position to take as an individual working in isolation or just from having listened to a lecture or seminar. Action learning sets help with the management of change and the development of leadership skills (see Table 7.2).

Table 7.2 Benefits of action learning

Individual practitioner	Organisation/clinical area
Greater breadth in understanding their organisation and building relationships necessary to take action	Shared knowledge and learning from wider range of colleagues.
More ability to analyse ambiguous data and solve complex problems	Enables effective action to be taken to creatively resolve difficult problems, to do things differently and improve continuously
Enhanced capacity to understand and initiate organisational changes	Organisational/clinical care change required as well as personal change
Increased focus on what makes a difference in a situation	More likely to develop leaders with a flexible, entrepreneurial approach (at all levels) who can manage change and uncertainty
Being more action focused and proactive in delivering results	Able to tackle difficult problems or when the organisation/clinical area faces crises, improving morale
Enhanced self-awareness and appreciation of personal impact on others, contributing to improved ability to work with others in teams	More cost effective than 'traditional' training courses and intimately linked to organisation/clinical area working
Developed flexibility in responding to changing situations and adapting a more flexible range of behaviour	Encourages effective teamwork, focuses and sustains the motivation of committed people and co-operation across internal organisational boundaries
Greater effectiveness in communicating proposals to senior managers	Offers an integrated path to personal and organisational learning at as fast a rate as the changes in the outside world

Organising the meetings for an action learning set

The first task of an action learning set is to agree the ground rules. Examples of a few ground rules for one action learning set are shown here.

Examples of ground rules for an action learning set

- All group members to agree that all discussions within the action learning set should remain confidential
- If something is discussed that an action-set member feels that they will have to take outside of the set (e.g. a code of conduct issue), this should be done with the agreement of the group

- All group members should be supportive to each other, as well as willing to challenge
- All participants should listen without interrupting and should actively listen, with no 'side-talking'
- There is no such thing as a 'stupid' question
- Make it fun
- These ground rules are to be referred to at the beginning of each meeting and are subject to revision by the group

Relationships are built up over time, and members care about projects succeeding. Either the facilitator or the group or both will agree how time available for the meeting will be divided so that each member gets a share of the time to focus on their own learning, or to contribute to a shared project. The action learning set looks at each issue in turn, analysing it using a critical incident/reflective process framework. Any actions identified should be recorded so that progress can be monitored. It is also useful if a record is made of key elements of the discussion; tasks and activities to be undertaken can then be signed up to in the form of an action plan.

Depending on the nature of the problem or project and the time scales, the action learning set will meet regularly with their facilitator, at mutually agreed times, dates and places, normally for around half a day. The set participants review progress, present recommendations, agree courses of action and evaluate results. There may be some shared preparation work to do between meetings. Everyone needs to honour these commitments if the set is to function effectively and complete its tasks.

Johnson and Johnson (1992) suggest that an effective co-operative learning group should contain five critical elements:

- positive interdependence – the trust among members that holds the group together
- interpersonal social skills – the ability to communicate with each other effectively
- reflection on group functioning and feeding this back to each other
- exchange of ideas and resources, promoting higher-level decision-making
- individual accountability, with all contributing to group accountability.

There is a constant and fascinating tension between the organising ability and facilitation skills of an outside facilitator and the team or community with which they are working. The facilitator is always in danger of 'helping' in a way that is not helpful because it is too controlling or because they fail to understand the situation, because they are an 'outsider'. The community is always in danger of irrationally rejecting the outsider or of becoming overly dependent. For these reasons, facilitators of action learning must follow frameworks for reflective practice and carefully monitor their facilitation practices (Kristiansen and Bloch-Poulsen, 2004).

It can be helpful if participants in an action-learning set prepare for set meetings by reading through their notes and recording their progress towards their action points beforehand. The set might agree to more elaborate forms of preparation, such as sending round forms with a synopsis of the work done since the last meeting. The group may invite brainstorming or force field analysis (factors hindering or facilitating a particular action plan) from the group, or present progress by a flipchart or handout, or simply hold an unstructured discussion. The following pro forma may be useful in aiding documentation.

Action Learning Set pro forma: Status report

Date . . . .   Time . . . .

What actions have I completed since the last meeting?

Action points outstanding:

What were the outcomes?

What is/are my most pressing problem(s)?

What do I want to achieve by the next meeting? Proposed next steps:

What could get in the way of achieving the next steps?

What do I want to get from the meeting?

Reflections of the meeting/feedback from group members:

- Successful action-learning groups call for non-judgemental attitudes, not imposing one's views or attitudes, asking questions rather than giving advice, and respecting the view of others.
- Action learning combines learning by taking action on real problems with learning from reflective self-assessment and review. Participants learn by diagnosing problems and devising solutions but also by making decisions and being responsible for achieving outcomes.
- Action learning sets often tackle crucial organisational problems for which there are no known answers. This involves participants moving beyond comfortable, familiar tasks to focus on how they respond to challenging, unfamiliar problems and will support innovation.
- Participants volunteer to tackle important problems that they want to have impact on and are willing to commit their time, energy and capabilities to resolving.
- Action learning focuses not only on how to tackle problems but also on the participant's own behaviour; strengths and development needs.
- Action learning offers opportunities to develop effective ways of working together and focus on teamwork and networking as well as the tasks.
- A facilitator can create the structure, process and the conditions for learning; providing both support and challenge; encouraging open feedback, questioning and encouraging exchanges of ideas or experiences. A facilitator can also provide a vital outside perspective on projects and personal development.
- Participants meet regularly during an agreed period of time to review progress and proposals to tackle difficulties, as well as to review their own learning, perceptions, behaviour and attitudes.

Peer learning

Peer learning involves peers learning from each other, and action-learning sets offer one method of encouraging peer learning. All of the people involved in peer learning should be equally dedicated to helping each other. For peer learning to be effective, the group needs to experience 'positive interdependence' (emphasising the importance and uniqueness of each person's efforts), face-to-face interaction and ensure that individual and group accountability are maintained.

Reflective activity

What experiences have you had in relation to peer learning? If it was successful think about why this was so. If it was not helpful, why was this?

How could you introduce peer learning into your current continuous professional development activities?

Peer learning extends beyond the task or project to develop leadership and relationship skills. Peer learning may, however, if poorly constructed, allow some team members to avoid fulfilling their team responsibilities. If the peer learning is part of the summative assessment, this particular problem, of individuals not taking on a suitable level of individual responsibility, can be minimised by including peer assessment of the individual performance of team members, as well as giving the group an overall assessment result. By asking for feedback from a peer, practitioners can learn about aspects of their practice of which they may not have been aware. Peer feedback can also build on self-assessment by providing greater awareness of strengths and opportunities for learning.

***

Key points **Top tips**

- Discuss incidents or examples from practice that illustrate your learning needs
- Ask peers to identify things that you do well in your practice as well as things that could enhance your practice
- Combine feedback from peers with your own self-assessment
- Choose peers who are familiar with your area of practice
- A peer does not have to come from the same professional group
- You can choose more than one peer to give you feedback
- A peer does not have to observe a practitioner's practice directly to be able to provide constructive feedback

***

Decision-making and action planning

Action and peer learning often take the form of working individually or together on a 'project'. A project can provide an important locus for learning (DeFillippi, 2001). Project work frequently leads participants along a 'journey through practice', where knowledge can be changed, shared, discarded or embedded. The article cited in the following Evidence base provides an example of a clinical setting undertaking a 'project'.

Evidence base

Take a look at Nolan, J. (2001) A flexible approach to Methicillin-Resistant Staphylococcus Aureus (MRSA). *Nursing Times*, **97**(46), 57–58.

Working in a surgical high-dependency unit with no specific area for isolation, prompted Joanne Leigh Nolan and her team to develop and implement guidelines for the management of patients with MRSA.

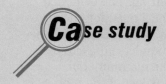

Case study

Knowledge underpinning practice decisions

Alex, an oncology specialist nurse, had to explain the various choices open to the woman with breast cancer. Alex was not sure whether she had really done the best for the patient, so that the woman was fully informed prior to making her treatment decision. Alex started to think about what had influenced her approach to patient communication. She had sat down with the patient and discussed the various oncology treatment options and had given the woman some information leaflets to take away to help her think things through. She had also given her contact telephone number so that, if the patient had any further points that needed clarifying, she could phone and ask. From past experience, Alex has come to see that patients understand and cope better with chemotherapy when they have it explained in this way. Various ways of explaining chemotherapy, including discussion alone, videos and the stories of other patients, had been tried previously, but, through 'trial and error' and watching other expert nurses in her past clinical working life, she determined that verbal discussion backed up with information leaflets was the 'best' approach. Based on what she felt intuitively would work with a particular patient and on non-verbal cues that she picked up, the way that Alex talked to each woman was different (not in content but style). Alex was also aware, through her post-registration studies, that the combination of verbal and written information leads to increased retention of the information and that patients informed in this way experience significantly less anxiety. Alex also made sure that she had the current evidence base, regarding the treatment regimens on offer, and had sought updating from journals and from other colleagues regarding the drugs available; she was also aware of her NHS Trust hospital's drug protocols for patients with this form of breast cancer.

Having read Alex's case study, identify the underlying reasons or 'source of knowledge' that she used to make her clinical decision.

Do you have any thoughts about her clinical reasoning?

In order to approach clinical decision-making in an 'evidence-based' way, you need to review the evidence available, thinking carefully and clearly about what makes most sense in influencing your clinical decisions. Evidence-based practice means integrating individual clinical expertise with the best available external evidence. There are advantages for health care professionals who practice in an evidence-based way as it means that their knowledge base continues improving and that they have increased confidence in their clinical decision-making. Research needs to be relevant to the clinical situation, acceptable to the professional and the patient, comprehensive, accurate, easily accessible, and understandable if nurses and other health care professionals are to implement the findings (Walsh and Wigens, 2003).

Evidence-based practice is a total process, which begins with knowing what clinical questions to ask and searching for relevant literature. Once all the relevant literature has been read and critically examined, this is shared and discussed with other clinical team members to find out whether they think it is relevant to practice. A comparison needs to be made between the 'best practice' identified through the literature search and the practice that currently exists, and thought given as to whether this 'best practice' is appropriate to the clinical setting. The evidence may support the previous practice, or there may be a need for change management. 'Old habits' can be hard to break so it is necessary for the whole team to 'own' the need for change, and action learning can be a useful route to ownership. The change needs to be maintained in practice over a reasonable time period. The final aspect of the process is the collation of evidence so that the impact of the change to practice can be assessed and evaluated (Walsh and Wigens, 2003).

Stages in the evidence-based practice process

1   Identify an area of practice
2   Undertake a literature review
3   Discuss the available literature with colleagues
4   Agree 'best practice' with colleagues
5   Compare 'best practice' to current practice
6   Make a change in practice if necessary
7   Evaluate the new practice

Whatever the scenario, effective action planning involves:

- breaking your goals down into smaller steps
- identifying the actions you need to take for each step
- considering how to overcome any constraints
- identifying people/resources that can help
- setting a target date for completion of each step
- trying to be realistic in the tasks you set yourself
- monitoring, reviewing and adapting the action plan on a regular basis.

Over to you

Think about a recent area of your practice where you or your clinical team had to action plan.

Ask yourself the following questions:

1   What result was I/were we trying to achieve?
2   What activities did I/we plan in order to achieve it?
3   Did I/we achieve the planned result?
4   If not, why not?
5   Did the activities make sense, in terms of what I/we were trying to achieve?
6   Could I/we have achieved the same result at less cost, spending less time, using fewer resources, with less strain on the people involved?
7   What would I/we do differently in future?
8   What have I learnt from this analysis?

When making a change in practice it is useful to have baseline information about the current practice to allow comparison when actions are taken, but do not just collect information for the sake of having it. You must have a purpose and a reason for collecting the information, particularly if other practitioners will be required to expend effort to help in the data collection. You need to focus your information-collection process around the questions that you want answered. Usually, when you are looking for evidence, it is to show progress in activities and to allow later comparison of efficiency, effectiveness and impact.

At the start of action planning, the questions to ask include:
- What sort of information do we need?
- How will we use the information?
- How can it be collected with the least possible trouble?
- Who will collect it?
- Who will analyse it?
- At the end of the delivery of the action plan, evaluation questions you might want to answer are:
  - How many?
  - How well?
  - How often?
  - Who benefited?
  - How did they benefit?

When you analyse the information, you are looking for the unexpected, and trying to learn from any deviations (differences from the expected) so that you can improve your practice.

Monitoring an action plan requires ongoing assessment of progress and can be done by the individuals involved, or people external to delivering the change can be asked to monitor progress: for example, a manager who is a stakeholder. Monitoring progress against action learning plans enables you to learn from mistakes and take corrective action when necessary. Once the goals of the action plan have been achieved, it is useful to evaluate the overall action planning process to identify learning.

Key points Top tips

- Many different forms of evidence can be used to inform clinical decisions and actions
- Effective action planning involves breaking down goals into smaller steps and considering how these can best be achieved
- It is useful to determine and collect baseline information prior to making a change to practice, so that, after the change has been implemented and when relevant information is collected, this can determine efficacy

This chapter has provided you with an understanding of a number of concepts that are related to experiential learning, such as peer, problem-based and action learning. As the discussion and examples of frameworks have shown, reflective practice can facilitate clinical decision-making, and the use of a range of evidence to inform practice is encouraged. I hope this chapter has provided you with some practical ways of starting reflective practice on your own, in pairs, or within groups.

RRRRRRapid recap

Check your progress so far by working through each of the following questions.

1   How does experiential learning differ from classroom-based traditional teaching?
2   List three frameworks that can guide reflection.
3   What are the stages of the adapted Gibbs' reflective cycle?
4   Define problem-based learning and action learning.
5   What stages are there in making an evidence-based change in practice?

If you have difficulty with one of these questions, read through the section again to refresh your understanding before moving on.

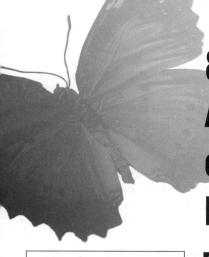

8
Assessment: using evidence to demonstrate learning through practice

Learning outcomes

By the end of this chapter you should be able to:

★ Explain the main aspects of the assessment of practice

★ Understand skills teaching and the linkage with assessment criteria

★ Appreciate how professional portfolios can provide evidence of improving clinical performance

★ Identify a range of evidence to utilise within practice

★ Explore the concept of expertise and the journey from novice to expert.

Introduction

Assessing another health care practitioner's practice is a privilege, and the learner is also privileged to receive the time and effort given to their assessment by a more experienced practitioner. To get the most from assessment, learners need to feel able to discuss their learning needs and be open to constructive feedback in the work setting. Much of the literature on the assessment of practice is concerned with what students should be learning and how to measure it. If the teaching methods used are experiential and focus on emulating professional practice, it is essential that practice assessment should be performance based, holistic, and allow learners to input their own decisions and solutions (Biggs, 2003). Assessment is crucial, as it greatly influences the curriculum and hence student learning (Ramsden, 1992). Strategic learners seek to maximise their chances of success by focusing their efforts on areas of their studies which contribute to their marks or grades (Kneale, 1997). Assessment of practice, it is argued, should encourage critical thinking, reflective practice and skills based on sound clinical knowledge.

Within this chapter we will take a look at practice assessment and the evidence that can be used to demonstrate that standards are being met. As portfolio-based continuous assessment is the most commonly used format, this will also be discussed. Novices increase their expertise through working in practice, and this is also addressed.

Assessment of practice

Put simply, assessment consists of finding out what and how much a person has learnt. There has been growing concern about the competence of health care professionals and the need to assess discrete skills, and this has led to the relocation of assessment into practice areas with clinical staff involvement. Assessment in practice encompasses a range of methods to measure a learner's competence to practise clinical skills and gives an assessor an opportunity to provide feedback, support and guidance.

It can be difficult to prepare practice assessors to ensure the reliable assessment of clinical skills, knowledge and attitudes. Validity is crucial, and, as Ramsden (1992) suggests, much assessment in higher education is flawed, owing to the widespread use of surface approaches where the student does not need to show an understanding of fundamental ideas. We need to ensure that mechanistic and reductionist approaches to assessment are avoided, so that the practice of nursing is not being reduced to a set of tasks or competences to be performed (Nicol and Freeth, 1998).

Assessment through observation in the work base is authentic, and interferes less with the ongoing service commitment of qualified staff (Simons and Parry-Crooke, 2001). Judgements regarding student competency are best made through observation, while standing nearby or a short distance away (Ohrling and Hallberg, 2001b). When students undertake complex tasks, they can be provided with hints before, during or after these nursing interventions from their mentors, but, if an emergency situation occurs, the student should step back to allow the experienced nurse to take over (Ohrling and Hallberg, 2001b). Previous clinical incidents can be discussed, and reflection on this, when combined with observation, is viewed as optimum for accurate assessment of practice.

Assessment is usually categorised as either formative or summative.

- **Formative assessment**. This takes place throughout the placement and is an informal assessment that helps to identify strengths and weaknesses and the level of student learning and progress. Formative assessment can be used to identify a need for further explanation, additional practice experience or whether learning can move on to other areas.

- **Summative assessment**. This usually takes place at the end of a placement and is a formal assessment where the 'mark' is used to determine the level of achievement. It determines how much has been learnt by the student and the extent to which the learning outcomes have been met.

The NMC (2005) states, 'Formative assessment is developmental and summative assessment is judgmental.' Registrants from any profession may be involved in formative assessment, but only NMC registrants should make summative judgements.

Separating assessment into 'assessment of theory' and 'assessment of practice' is artificial and does not help the student practitioner. Contemporary assessment encompasses practice and theory, as well as summative and formative elements, and this is often facilitated through learning contracts and personal portfolios (Jasper 1996).

Mentors and assessors have the following responsibilities regarding assessment:

- to maintain high personal standards of practice, teaching and assessment
- to determine the standard of care delivery of learners, and to make professional judgements about student performance from this
- to actively contribute to what is taught, learnt and assessed within clinical practice.

Teaching and assessing a skill

Being unable to perform procedures competently is stressful for a novice practitioner, so students are keen to develop skills. Skills can range from carrying out practical tasks (e.g. assisting with hygiene needs), to assessing patients (e.g. taking observations and interpreting these), to communicating (e.g. breaking bad news). Clinical skill laboratories, objective structured clinical examinations (OSCE) and manikins are increasingly being used to allow students to learn and assess skills in a safe environment, as it is not always practicable or ethical for some skills to be learnt initially in a clinical setting. However, such methods can only assist to a limited extent and students need to try out new skills with patients in clinical settings.

There are three main stages to teaching a skill:

1 Sensitising students to the skill

   (They should be able to:

   - understand why the skill is important to them, both in the context of the course and in professional practice
   - analyse the skill in terms of its constituent parts
   - distinguish good practice from poor
   - evaluate the effectiveness of the skill when demonstrated)

2 Facilitating practice in the skill

3 Giving feedback on the performance of the skill.

Skills have been 'broken down' by Fisher *et al.* (2005) to incorporate reflections on skill development:

- a definition/explanation of what it is you are trying to do (what is it?)
- a rationale for the skill you are performing (why do it?)
- what you need to know in order to do it (knowledge underpinning practice)
- how to do it
- sources of information (reference list)
- reflection on how you did.

In the past, skills development was sometimes described as 'see one, do one and then teach one', but a preferred approach involves the supervisor breaking the demonstration of skills process into manageable steps. These steps can be:

1 **Demonstration** – the supervisor demonstrates skills at normal speed without any commentary.

2 **Deconstruction** – the supervisor demonstrates with an accompanying commentary.

3 **Comprehension** – the supervisor demonstrates with an accompanying commentary from the learner.

4 **Performance** – the learner demonstrates giving an accompanying commentary (Peyton, 1998).

Teaching a skill is linked to a judgement as to whether the learner can perform the skill adequately and a discussion about how the skill may be altered by differing circumstances. Using this approach to skill development encourages the student to move from 'consciously incompetent' to 'consciously competent', as shown in the 'Learning a skill' matrix (Howell and Fleishman, 1982). Practice is the single most effective way to move from stages 3 to 4 in the matrix. The assessor can assess competence (can the student undertake this skill safely in a supervised environment?) and performance (are they able to practice this alone safely?).

Awareness

1. **Unconsciously incompetent**	2. **Consciously incompetent**
• the person is not aware that they have a particular deficiency in the area concerned • the person is not aware of the existence or relevance of the skill area	• the person is aware of their deficiency in this area, ideally through attempting or trying to use the skill • the person has a measure of the extent of their deficiency in the relevant skill, and a measure of what level of skill is required for their own competence
4. **Unconsciously competent**	3. **Consciously competent**
• the skill is so practised that it becomes 'second nature' • might now be able to teach others the skill concerned	• the person can perform the skill reliably at will • the person needs to concentrate and think in order to perform the skill

Practice

Figure 8.1 Learning a skill matrix (after Howell and Fleishman, 1982)

Steinaker and Bell (1979) developed an experiential learning taxonomy that is often used, sometimes in an adapted form, to assess the level of practice learning and skills achieved by a learner. This consists of:

1 **Exposure** – the student has observed the skill being performed by a competent practitioner

2 **Participation** – the student has assisted a competent practitioner in the performance of the skill

3 **Identification** – the student has performed the skill under the supervision of a registered practitioner

4 **Internalisation** – the student has sustained a skilled performance in a variety of settings under the supervision of a registered practitioner

5 **Dissemination** – the student has maintained professional competence and has enabled others to develop their knowledge and skills.

An example of how this might be used in assessing the ability to administer drugs is given here.

Assessing the level of experiential learning (after Steinaker and Bell, 1979)

1 Exposure – the learner is introduced to the experience and is conscious of it as an observer. They should be able to describe some of the underpinning knowledge (The implication is that the learner is not safe to participate as yet, even with supervision.)

'I watch another giving a patient their drugs.'

2 Participation – the learner has made a decision to become part of the experience, and participates under direct observation. (They may need prompting and guidance, and have a basic understanding of underpinning knowledge.)

'I administer drugs under close supervision.'

3 Identification – the learner identifies with the experience both intellectually and emotionally and is able to undertake care under supervision, but may require some guidance (is usually confident, safe and effective and able to discuss the application of knowledge).

'I can competently administer drugs, although I still require them to be checked.'

4 Internalisation – the learner's experience affects their behaviours and the way they do things, and they have the capacity to perform their practice with minimal guidance (is competent, safe and effective, and is able to demonstrate applied and situated knowledge).

'Administering drugs is something I do most days when working clinically.'

5 Dissemination – the learner is now able to confidently execute skilled practice, to express the experience and advocate for others. They can also influence and teach others.

'I am skilful in drug administration and supervise and teach this to other staff and students.'

The criteria for assessment of performance should be clearly stated and specific, and high standards should be encouraged but these do need to be attainable. Students and assessors are often asked to assess the achievement of specified learning outcomes. The term 'learning outcome' encompasses what it is that a learner can do, what they understand, and what personal qualities and attributes they have as a result of their learning.

Assessment criteria for a competency can be specified using three domains of learning:

- the cognitive domain – knowledge outcomes (concerned with the acquisition of knowledge (how we acquire information and what we need to know)
- the psychomotor domain – performance outcomes (relating to the development of skills and 'doing')
- the affective domain – attitudes and values displayed (formation of beliefs, values and attitudes).

Example of a learning outcome

By the end of the placement, the learner will be able to care for patients and relatives at times when they appear dissatisfied with an aspect of their care.

Knowledge outcomes

- Discuss the stages of dealing with patient and relative dissatisfaction from an informal response to a formal complaint.
- Describe the policies, guidance and role of the Patient Advice and Liaison Service (PALS) and Complaints Service.
- Discuss evidence available regarding patient satisfaction and dissatisfaction.

Performance outcomes

- Support and communicate effectively with patients and relatives who are dissatisfied with an aspect of care.
- Refer to PALS and Complaints colleagues where appropriate.
- Identify ways of improving satisfaction with patient care, informed by patient feedback.

Attitude and values

- Be empathetic and show respect towards patients and relatives who are dissatisfied with care.
- Appreciate good patient feedback, and recognise poor patient communication.
- Take a balanced and professional approach to all those involved in a complaints procedure.

Assessment criteria might be:

- The learner uses a polite and confident approach in all communications.
- The learner is able to decide rapidly whether they can manage the area of dissatisfaction with care in an appropriate manner, or whether they need to refer to a qualified practitioner.
- The learner is able to identify the route by which patients can access staff who can give advice on initiating a formal complaint.
- The learner is able to use evidence to inform changes to improve patient satisfaction with care.

Assessment criteria need to be easily related to learning outcomes. Evidence for the example on page 148 could be obtained through direct observation (e.g. watching the learner handle a dissatisfied patient), discussion (e.g. questioning and discussion about how a particular situation was/could be handled) and written information (e.g. reflective account in a learning journal, diary of a visit to PALS or the Complaints department). No single procedure is adequate for assessing clinical competence, so in the last example the more continuous the process of gaining evidence of achievement of the learning outcomes, the greater the predictive validity (Oliver and Endersby, 2000).

Developing assessment criteria that help assessors to discern the level of practice, and that are easy to use, can be a problem. Pfeil (2003) suggests that involving practitioners, mentors and lecturers in devising assessment criteria results in improved criteria for the summative assessment of practice.

Biggs (2003) argues that criterion-referenced assessment, rather than norm-referenced, should be adopted and there should be a more holistic and divergent approach, involving significant peer and self-assessment.

Norm referencing can occur even when clear criteria are available for assessment judgements. Practitioners who work regularly with students encounter a variety of students and comzparison of those who are at the same stage of training is difficult to avoid. Acknowledging that this can happen is the first step in reducing a 'norm-referencing effect'. If a mentor has recently worked with a second-year student who they perceived as excellent, the next second-year student on this placement may have their assessment compromised unless the mentor ensures that they assess using the explicit criteria provided by the education institute (criteria referencing).

A pass/fail criterion for practice can be easier to use, as all that is required is to discriminate between safe and unsafe practice. Grading and banding require assessors to use criteria to discriminate between varying levels of practice and to reward excellence, although there can be a 'central tendency error' with the bulk of the marks falling into the middle grade or band (Quinn, 1995).

Andre (2000) advocates graded assessment because it can clarify for students the minimal competency requirements and also describe and record meritorious practice. An example of assessment criteria is given overleaf in Table 8.1.

Table 8.1 Example of Diploma Level practice criteria

Grade	Criteria
70% +	Care actions are always safe, appropriate and effective. Practice is always based on evidence from research/literature (where available). Beginning to act as a role model and influencing others through supervision of their learning Beginning to disseminate aspects of their practice Able to evaluate practice of self and others Often proactive in care actions Demonstrates the ability to link ethical, social and political actions to patient care and nursing practice within the setting Utilises developed skills within the clinical area
60–69%	Care actions are always safe, appropriate and effective. Practice is always based on evidence from research/literature (where available). Beginning to influence the practice of others Able to evaluate changing clinical situations and to sometimes supervise the learning and development of others Sometimes proactive in care actions Demonstrates awareness of the links between ethical, social and political actions Utilises developing skills within the clinical area
50–59%	Care actions are always safe, appropriate and effective. Practice is always based on evidence from research/literature (where available). Recognises change within practice situations Identifies with the area of practice Demonstrates awareness of the broader links between ethical, social and political structures and the context of nursing practice Skills are developing, but continues to need supervision
40–49%	Care actions are always safe, appropriate and effective. Practice is often, but not always, based on evidence from research/literature (where available). Beginning to reflect on the relationships between principles and practice Demonstrates awareness of the broader links between ethical, social and political structures and the context of nursing practice Further skills development required
Referral 39% or less	Care actions are not always appropriate and effective. Practice is often not based upon evidence from research/literature (where available). Practice is rules-based, reflecting a lack of self-awareness and the ability to evaluate the clinical environment Demonstrates limited awareness of the broader links between ethical, social and political structures and the context of nursing practice Further skills development is required

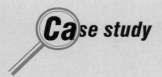 *Case study*

Assessing practice using grading criteria

Karen, an experienced mentor, is supervising three student nurses on clinical placement. When asked to outline the key features of their current level of practice to the link lecturer she describes them in the following way:

1   Grace is coming to the end of year one of her nurse training. She is a mature student who had a number of years' experience as a health care assistant prior to starting her nursing studies. She has good levels of practical skills and is hard working and able to use her initiative beyond that of many nurses at this stage of their course. Karen has noticed that Grace can be rather abrupt with patients who

are quite dependent and sometimes seems to be concentrating on the task whilst excluding other aspects of care, such as her communication and her nurse–patient relationship development. When Karen asks Grace to discuss the underpinning rationale for her care, Grace says, 'I did it because I was asked to.'

2   Jack is an adult branch student of nursing at the end of his second year of studies. He appears to be rather hesitant in his delivery of care, and comes over as shy and nervous. He talks about his motivation to learn, but rarely uses his initiative and requires a lot of direction from Karen about what he is expected to achieve whilst on this placement. He is reliable in his work and has sound basic care skills. When questioned about what knowledge underpins his practice, Jack shows a sound understanding of the rationales for care.

3   Meena is near to the end of her third year of nurse training. She is a bright and energetic student, although sometimes she is a little immature in her discussions with colleagues and she has been reticent in identifying her personal learning needs. Meena has developed high-level clinical skills, shows motivation to learn and is sensitive to patient needs. She has needed considerable encouragement to display leadership skills, needing much prompting to undertake patient handovers, and gives succinct but insufficiently detailed reports of her observations.

Using the grading criteria for assessment of practice shown in Table 8.1, how do you think Karen would assess these three students' level of practice?

Looking at her accounts of the students, can you spot any potential risks in Karen's undertaking criterion-referenced assessment using these grading criteria?

Jasper and Fulton (2005) suggest that while portfolios have been used for some years in health care to assess professional attainment, the assessment process and criteria have mainly been rudimentary and underdeveloped. The criteria on which assessment is based are often locally developed, open to varying interpretations and adapted from existing higher education criteria, which are academically based, such as the Quality Assurance Agency for Higher Education's generic outcomes expected at different levels of academic study (QAAHE, 2001).

Table 8.2 Example of Masters level practice assessment marking criteria (Jasper and Fulton, 2005)

The portfolio should demonstrate achievement of the following:
A critical and systematic understanding of a specialist knowledge base
Originality in utilising knowledge base and methods of inquiry in practice
The ability to assess complex situations and articulate problems
Decision-making and professional judgement in planning strategies to deal with complex situations
The ability to act autonomously in planning and implementation and use others appropriately
The development of new insights which enhance and develop practice
Independent, critical and reflective thinking
Effective communication with professionals and non-professionals
Personal insight and self–awareness, acknowledgement of own limitations
Presentation of the portfolio within a coherent structure, which contains all the required elements, including the use of English and referencing system

Assessment of practice criteria is used for vocational as well as higher education health care courses. Assessment and accreditation criteria in National Vocational Qualifications (NVQs) are derived from a functional analysis of an occupational area (Ecclestone, 1996), and these functions are broken down into units of competence and then into elements within these units. Elements of competence are assessed using performance criteria incorporating a requirement for the range and scope of situations and underpinning knowledge.

Assessment criteria within vocational awards have defined standards and indicate the quality of evidence that learners must demonstrate in order to achieve the learning outcomes. Evidence of the achievement of an element of competence is collected either directly (through observation of workplace activity) or indirectly. Indirect demonstration of competence can take the form of:

- care records
- testimonial evidence
- simulations and role-play
- work-based assignments and projects
- answers to questions
- test results.

NVQ evidence is assessed by work-based assessors who determine if the person is competent or not yet competent and needs to generate further practice and development skills and additional evidence. Once the work-based assessor deems the person to be competent, the unit responsible for NVQs can ensure that the evidence is internally verified (checked for consistent marking) and, following this, externally verified.

Whether the course is vocationally or higher-education based, Jarvis and Gibson (1997) describe five basic requisites for assessing students:

1 look
2 listen
3 listen
4 discuss
5 decide.

First, the assessor observes the learner when working with him or her. The assessor needs to be aware of the learner's actions and use their observations to inform their future teaching. The assessor also needs to listen to what the learner says to him or her and to what others (patients, colleagues and other members of the multidisciplinary team) in the learning environment say. The observations and listening can then contribute to discussion concerning elements of practice, particularly those that cannot be observed; careful use of questioning can also ascertain assessment information (Open University, 2001). The discussion can also relate to written evidence from the learner, such as reflective accounts. A conclusion has then to be reached as a result of the four previous processes.

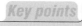

Top tips

When assessing clinical performance:

- Identify skills to be assessed
- Know what you would expect from a student at different stages in their programme, but make sure that you assess in line with the criteria
- Structure your working with a student to allow you to observe skills and behaviour as often as possible
- Gather information from a range of sources, e.g. student, other colleagues, patients
- Offer timely and constructive feedback
- Get students to discuss their rationales for their care

Issues affecting the assessment process

As assessing practice is a complex activity, the practice aspect of a course has often been separated from the academic achievement and awarded only a pass or fail grade, even though many professional bodies require practice to have equal value to theory. Phillips *et al.* (2000b) found that in some scenarios assessment was viewed as a necessary but irksome 'bolt-on' activity.

To have validity, assessment should test what it is designed to test: therefore, the ability to administer drugs safely could not be assessed by questioning or discussion alone; it would require observation of drug administration undertaken by the student. For assessment to have reliability, different assessors should give similar scores for the same demonstration of care delivery, and summative assessment should relate to consistent performance. So, in the example of drug administration, if one mentor deems the student safe and effective in their drug administration, this should also be the case if another mentor witnesses this student's drugs' management on the same occasion.

Reflective activity

Think about two occasions, one when you felt you were unfairly assessed and one where you felt fairly assessed. In each case, what factors led you to this viewpoint? Did the incident where you felt you were unfairly assessed affect your future learning?

Continuous assessment of practice is seen as being more representative than 'one-off' assessment, where factors such as ill health and anxiety can adversely affect the outcome. Continuous assessment through portfolio assessment is more likely to motivate deep learning (Tiwari and Tang, 2003) and can include evidence of the demonstration of skills and knowledge in practice, an analysis of a critical incident, or a reflection on actual practice. However, continuous assessment takes time and energy, and protected time should be allocated and prioritised for 'assessment-only' activities (Phillips *et al.*, 2000b). Portfolio assessment also allows for the existence of unintended learning (Biggs, 2003). McMullan *et al.* (2003) suggest that portfolio assessment should contain a case made by the learner as to how the prescribed outcomes have been attained, and evidence should be offered to support this case.

Issues to be addressed in assessing portfolios include:

- validity and reliability (does the evidence accurately match the performance criteria and assess the things it claims to assess? – requires unambiguous wording of criteria and careful preparation of assessors)

- inter-rater moderation (when sampled, is there consistency in approach and how is this feedback to assessors maintained?)

- subjectivity (are the purpose and expectations clarified before assessing the work?)

- evidence usage (is the evidence generated the learner's own work, and is there enough to infer competence? Is there guidance/guidelines on evidence use for students and assessors?)

- reflective writing (do the assessment criteria guide the level of reflection for students and assessors?)

- marking criteria (do the assessment criteria require and help in differentiating between excellent, good, adequate and failing work in a consistent way?).

Although assessment criteria assist objectivity, there are common pitfalls in the assessment process, which place validity and reliability at risk. Students' learning during clinical placements is, to a large extent, affected by the perceptions of assessors and students. Assessment that is based on discrete assessed episodes, such as an aseptic technique procedure, creates high anxiety levels and has a negative 'backwash' effect (Alderson and Wall, 1993). This type of assessment requires only lower-level cognition, such as factual recall or reproduction of a skill.

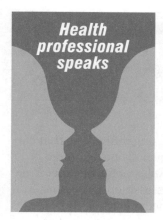

Health professional speaks

Student

I was quite concerned that I wouldn't get all of my competencies signed off. There were only a few shifts left to work with my mentor. The assessment dictated what I learnt on the ward. . . at times. I even gave up the chance of going to the endoscopy unit with one of the patients to observe a procedure, because it was not a priority to achieve in my assessment of practice learning outcomes.

The 'halo' effect occurs when the student is judged with regard to their popularity (Quinn, 1995). The concept that a 'good nurse' is synonymous with a 'nice person' continues in the minds of some assessors. It can be difficult for an assessor to decide that a student nurse has not met the assessment criteria when many of the clinical team have commented on what a nice, friendly team member he or she is.

Reflective activity

Accountability in assessment: within your professional career, there is likely to have been a time when you have expressed the thought that a person should never have qualified (his or her attitudes or skills are appalling). What reasons might explain how this professional practitioner was allowed to qualify? How could you in your professional role prevent this situation from occurring?

A positive backwash effect involves students demonstrating a personal interpretation of the underlying principles of their practice and a deeper approach to learning. An assessor's open questioning technique can create higher-level discussion and, by focusing on what the learner does not know, can promote thinking and problem solving. A supportive environment, where people can say, 'I don't know', helps with this. Biggs (2003) argues that a positive backwash effect can be facilitated if the assessment reflects the learning goals, so in clinical practice this could be for students to develop a variety of clinical skills, to understand the knowledge informing patient care, and to acclimatise to the professional community of practice. This form of authentic clinical assessment asks students to demonstrate their competence to think, decide and act in the reality of clinical practice.

Evidence base

Read: Wallace, B. (2003) Practical issues of student assessment. *Nursing Standard*, **17**(31), 33–36.

Student health care professionals may have learning difficulties that can affect their assessment. Mentors and assessors usually have limited knowledge of how to assist students who have dyslexia, for instance, and if not recognised this can lead to considerable assessment problems. Although this book can only offer limited guidance regarding this, perhaps the most important advice for students and mentors is that a confidential discussion early on in the placement can reduce the potential for problems within the assessment period.

Key points **Top tips**

When helping students who have told you that they have dyslexia:

- Provide pre-placement information using Arial fonts (as these are easier to read)
- Ask them what their main difficulties are, and how you can help them
- Ask questions clearly and concisely
- Offer demonstrations and give clear instructions that are carefully sequenced
- Allow practice in recording patient documentation prior to requiring the student to contribute entries to patient records, and countersign all entries
- Give time to independently calculate drug dosages, and always check these

Evidence base

Take a look at the following websites:
British Dyslexia Association www.bdadyslexia.org.uk
National Bureau for students with disabilities www.skill.co.uk

When student learning is taking place, the mentor is responsible for ensuring that preparation is sufficient not to put patients at risk, and that confidentiality is maintained within any documentation contained in assessment portfolios. Valid assessment can be put at risk if the mentor's role as a confidence-builder is given precedence over giving unfavourable feedback. A degree of self-reported working by a student or testimonial evidence is acceptable, but this should not form the basis of the overall assessment decision. Practitioners who have been adequately prepared for the assessment role should have confidence in their individual assessment judgements, in the same way that they make confident decisions about client care. As students move through different clinical placements they are being assessed by many practitioners and, collectively, this process should reduce concerns about the overall subjectivity of the assessment process for a student on a registered professional course.

Using evidence

Continuous assessment of practice often means that a portfolio of practice evidence is gathered to show achievement of the learning outcomes. A portfolio can be simply a tangible record of what someone has done, or a purposeful collection of materials that communicates a practitioner's development. McMullan *et al.* (2003) conducted a comprehensive literature review on the use of portfolios to assess holistic competence (including knowledge, skills, attitudes, performances and levels of sufficiency). A holistic way of viewing competence in portfolio assessment can help to overcome criticisms that assessment of competence can be fragmented, ignores context, lacks objectivity, and fails to assess knowledge, skills and attitudes in a comprehensive manner.

Scholes *et al.* (2004) looked at how mentors and nursing students match learning outcomes and competencies to their practice and then reconstruct experiences into the format required for the documentation within a portfolio. Portfolios enable assessors to measure student learning, help encourage reflective thinking, critical analytical skills, self-directed learning and provide detailed evidence of a practitioner's competence. To achieve maximum benefit from the portfolio there has to be a fit between the portfolio framework and the professional practice that is to be assessed (Scholes *et al.*, 2004). By engaging in a mentored, co-operative, and reflective process of portfolio development, students are able formatively to develop their self-assessment skills, make sense of what they were doing and plan their continuous improvement.

Endacott *et al.* (2004) identified four main forms of portfolio:

1   The shopping trolley – evidence is placed into a file with little structure and may include photocopies of articles and teaching notes, and resembles a resource file.

2   The toast rack – evidence is organised and slotted in under learning outcomes, but there is a large collection of papers, again including photocopied articles.

3   The spinal column model –uses competencies or learning outcomes to structure the portfolio, with the evidence being

inserted behind each learning outcome and combined with a
reflective commentary.

4   The cake mix model – this is a reflective commentary that asks the
learner to show how and what they have achieved and learnt and
how the evidence supports this.

Models 3 (spinal column) and 4 (cake mix) are most appropriate for
health care professional education. Jasper and Fulton (2005) suggest
that a general rule should be that the only evidence included should be
referenced within a reflective review or a case should be made with
regard to the learning outcomes. I also agree with Jasper and Fulton
(2005) when they say that quality is more important than quantity in
portfolio evidence.

Over to you

Here is a list of methods of evidencing practice assessment that could
be used within a portfolio. Identify which ones you have come across. Find out
about those you have not been involved with before, and decide if these could be
used within your future practice. The methods are:

- observation of practical skills
- student self assessment
- discussion
- learning contracts
- guided study
- written reflection
- testimony of others
- interviews
- patient comments and feedback
- peer evaluation
- audit or data collection
- case study
- team project.

The mentor who is observing a learner is also an active participant in the
clinical setting. It is easy for both the mentor and the learner to get
carried away with delivering patient care in a clinical context, so much
so that sometimes both can forget to record assessment evidence until a
great deal later, which might reduce the richness and accuracy of the
feedback. Observation is a powerful way to assess the practice of
learners, giving an opportunity to observe learners at work and to
compare this with what they say about their practice. It can be

particularly motivating for a student to receive overt praise for exceptional practice, and the praise can be reinforced through written assessment records or testimonial statements. As the mentor observes, they progressively focus their attention on any issues that have started to emerge. Just watching and working alongside a student can be enough on which to base an assessment decision; however, it can be useful to triangulate this evidence by assessing understanding through discussion with the learner.

Over to you

Choosing and using evidence in a portfolio: think of a piece of evidence you have within your portfolio. Ask yourself the following questions about this piece of evidence.

1   What experience and knowledge do I already have and can demonstrate from this piece of evidence?
2   What are the implications professionally?
3   What practical examples can I give to demonstrate my skills and competence to support this evidence?
4   What other sources of evidence can I draw on to inform this section of my portfolio?
5   What literature could support this evidence?
6   How can I demonstrate best practice from this piece of evidence?
7   What ongoing/further development could I identify from this?

Not all the questions will be appropriate for each piece, but asking these makes you consider the reasons why you are including it and what other complementary evidence should be added.

When included within portfolios, discussions and the narrative accounts of practice allow assessors to examine specific and individual learning, rather than a more general, abstract discussion of practice.

Evidence base

Obtain the following article and read the account of using reflective learning journals.

Thorpe, K. (2004) Reflective learning journals: from concept to practice. *Reflective Practice*, **5**(3), 1–18.

Keeping a learning journal to inform reflective writing and narratives necessitates taking 'time out' from a busy day or dedicating time at the end of the day, but does allow the writer to figure out their learning. A learning journal is a record, enabling the learner to review, analyse, inform decision-making and action plan. Students are responsible for keeping their assessment of practice documentation during their placement, but should make this available whenever required by the mentor. One way of reviewing reflective learning accounts is offered here to assist those developing reflective evidence, as well as those who are responsible for assessment.

Assessment indicators for reflective work (adapted from Moon, 1999)

Purpose

- The student should demonstrate understanding of the purpose, selection and description of the issues on which they reflect.

Description of an event or issue

- Description is present and provides an adequate focus for reflection.
- Description includes statement of observations, comments on personal behaviour, comments on reactions/feelings, comments on context.

Additional information

- Relevant knowledge, theory, experience and feelings.
- Suggestions from others.
- New information.
- Other factors e.g. ethical, moral, political and contextual.

Reflective thinking

- Able to structure the material – was an identified reflective framework used?
- Was theory linked to practice?
- The viewing of issues/events from different points of view.
- Evidence of new ideas being tested in practice or revisited and revised.

A conclusion

- A statement of either what has been learnt, solved or actions that relate to the incident or area of practice.
- Identification of a new area for further reflection.

As suggested by Goodman (1989), another way of reviewing reflections on practice is to determine the level of the reflection using the factors outlined in Table 8.3.

Table 8.3 Assessing levels of reflection (adapted from Goodman, 1989)

Level 1	Reflection to reach given objectives: Criteria are limited to issues of efficiency, effectiveness and accountability.
Level 2	Reflection on the relationship between principles and practice. There is an assessment of the implications, consequences and rationale for actions and beliefs.
Level 3	Reflection incorporates all of the above and in addition ethical and political concerns. Deliberations over the value of professional practice are included and the practitioner makes links between the practice setting and broader social structures.

A difficult aspect of working in health care is acknowledging your own beliefs and values and recognising that they may be very different from the beliefs and values held by your clients or patients and your peers. Reflective writing within a portfolio allows you to explore your professional values and beliefs. However, Orland-Barak and Wilhelem (2005) found that some nursing students used procedural professional language in their accounts of their learning, concentrating their narratives on describing biomedical care procedures, such as changing a colostomy bag, with rarely any deeper-level reflection being offered. This focus is understandable from a 'novice' perspective where skill performance is often a priority. Orland-Barak and Wilhelem (2005) take the view that it is important to allow student nurses time to look at the instrumental aspects of practice, as this is a novice's starting point for making sense of practice. Novices have been characterised as concrete in their thinking, using this form of reasoning because initially they need to adopt a single perspective on a problem before they can learn sensitivity to varying contexts. Mentors should allow students time to work on these fragmented aspects of practice, whilst encouraging them to transform these procedural and instrumental ways of thinking about practice into integrated personal and professional reflections.

Work-place learning has become increasingly valued, for instance the accreditation of prior experiential learning (APEL). Challis (1993) suggests that the fundamental principle of accreditation of prior (experiential) learning is that learning through experience is capable of gaining recognition and credit, regardless of the time, place and context where it is achieved, and is not dependent on any formal setting.

- Accreditation of prior learning can be matched to the learning outcomes that can be gained through formal qualification, with learners seeking 'credit' for showing how their experiential learning matches that of the qualification.
- The outcomes from prior certificated learning can be matched to outcomes of a formal qualification in order to gain exemption from particular modules.

- Accreditation of prior learning can be used as an alternative entry qualification to join a programme (termed 'advanced standing').

It is rare, however, for an entire qualification to be formed through the basis of past achievements alone. Evidence used in assessing prior learning may be direct (e.g. reflective writing, teaching plans, assignments, projects, articles) or indirect (e.g. certificates or witness testimonies).

Macdonald and Savin-Baden (2004) advocate that assessment of learners should ideally:

- be based in a practice context in which students will find themselves working in the future

- assess what the professional does in their practice, which is largely process-based professional activity, underpinned by appropriate knowledge, skills and attitudes

- reflect the learner's development from a novice to an expert

- encourage learners to appreciate and experience the fact that in a professional capacity they will encounter patients, clients, users, professional bodies and peers, who will continue to 'assess' them

- engage learners in self-assessment and reflection as the basis for future continuing professional development and self-directed learning

- consider the extent to which assessment practices are inclusive or whether they discriminate against certain students.

Novice to expert

Assessing practice evidence can help in determining the level of practice working. Benner (1984) identified the 'journey' that students take from being novices (students) to expert practitioners, and how nurses uncover and create knowledge through actual experiences. She built on the work of Dreyfus and Dreyfus (1979) and their model of skill acquisition developed through researching trainee aircraft pilots, which produced five levels of proficiency in the movement of novice to expert. Benner (1984) interviewed beginning nurses and expert nurses who had both been involved in the same situations, and examined both forms of narrative. An interpretative approach was then used to analyse the data, taking into account the context and the meaning that they made of the situation. Benner (1984) found that the key to expert practice was the ability to 'experience nursing' and then to integrate this into existing and new knowledge. The five levels of proficiency identified by Benner are outlined here.

Levels of proficiency (after Benner, 1984)

1 Novice – have had no experience of the situation; may show rigid adherence to taught rules and plans, little situational perception, no discretionary judgement

2 Advanced Beginner – demonstrates marginally acceptable performance, using guidelines for action, based on attributes or aspects; situational perceptions still limited; all attributes and aspects are treated separately and given equal importance

3 Competent – has been in similar situations and begins to see his or her actions in terms of the 'bigger' picture; coping with many forms of information, sees actions partly in terms of long-term goals, conscious planning, standardised and routinised procedures

4 Proficient – perceives situations as a whole and demonstrates a 'smooth' clinical performance; sees what is most important in a situation, perceives deviations from the normal, decision-making less laboured

5 Expert – no longer relying on principles, rules or guidelines to connect their actions to the appropriate situation; intuitive grasp of situations based on tacit understanding, analytical approaches only used in novel situations or where problems occur, has a vision of what is possible

At each stage of development, there is progress in three different aspects of skilled performance. The learner moves from a reliance on abstract principles to using past concrete experiences as paradigms; from seeing the situation as a set of equally important bits to seeing it as a complete whole (where only some parts are relevant); and from being an observer in the situation to being thoroughly engaged.

Over to you

Accompany someone you recognise as an 'expert' in clinical practice during a clinical episode or patient interaction. The 'expert' and you have different viewpoints on this care episode. Spend time discussing what they and you think happened. The content and learning from the clinical episode is more easily visualised as you are talking about the clinical care close to the event.

What did the other practitioner do differently compared with what you would have done in the management of the clinical episode or care delivery?

Students benefit from sustained working alongside qualified practitioners. Ebright *et al.* (2004), who studied novice 'near miss' and adverse events, concluded that support for novice nurses in acute care environments should include consistent and available expertise. Workloads can be very unpredictable and experts can recognise risk and intervene prior to errors occurring, and expectations of novices need to be managed, even up to a year post-registration.

Benner (1984) advocated that novices should work alongside experts but elaborated little on what methods should be used to optimise learning through practice. Rogoff (1990) suggests that mentors and clinical supervisors can help novices with difficult problems by structuring sub-goals from the problem, focusing their learning on manageable aspects such as a certain skill required. Lauder *et al.* (2003) stress the significance of developing a 'reservoir' of knowledge and experience of particular cases so that the novice nurse builds a 'cognitive library' of nursing information for practice.

> ### Over to you
>
> Examine the assessment tool used within the local health care practitioner education programme. Is there anything about this programme which appears to be based on Benner's model or any of the other level descriptors discussed here? If not, how might you find out about the underpinning knowledge that informed the development of this assessment tool?

Determining expertise can be difficult. A concept analysis of the term 'expertise' (Manley and McCormack, 1997) identified:

- the attributes of holistic practice knowledge, knowing the patient, **saliency**, **moral agency** and **skilled know-how**
- the enabling factors of reflective ability, organisation of practice, interpersonal relationships, autonomy and authority, and recognition by others.

The Royal College of Nursing Expertise in Practice project (Manley *et al.*, 2005) found that expertise, supported by critical reflective abilities, allowed experts to deconstruct their professional knowledge and artistry, but that this could also bring increased frustration with workplace constraints. Nurses with expertise were able to offer knowledgeable individualised care, using intuition, caring and empathy. 'Experts' were able to adapt and alter standard procedures and to change practice, where necessary, to meet the needs of service and patients, and their commitment to sharing their expertise was recognised by peers (Manley *et al.*, 2005).

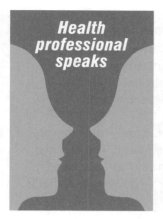

Patient: identifying expertise

Paul has such a calm, approachable way with him that you genuinely believe him when he says, 'Give me a phone if you have any worries'. I know he must be really busy, but when you speak to him he gives you his full attention. He has so much knowledge about my problem and is very skilled, and he understands what this disease means to me. He helps me to navigate all the different departments that are involved in my care, and everyone who he works with thinks really highly of him. He's very professional without being 'stand-offish'.

Critical thinking is an essential component of professional accountability and quality nursing care, and critical thinkers exhibit confidence, contextual perspective, creativity, flexibility, inquisitiveness, intellectual integrity, intuition, open-mindedness, perseverance, and reflection (Scheffer and Rubenfeld, 2000). Staib (2003) found that reflection, creativity, contextual perspective, and open-mindedness were the most common critical-thinking 'habits of the mind' addressed within nursing programmes and that, despite widespread interest in and recognition of the importance of developing critical-thinking skills, it was difficult to achieve.

Professional portfolios

The professional portfolio is considered to be one medium for expressing expertise, critical thinking and the progression from novice to expert. Health care professionals have to provide evidence of their competence and professional development to patients, their statutory bodies and their employer. The portfolio can illustrate all the elements needed for giving high-quality care and prove professional competence from multiple sources, such as work in practice, reflection, literature, formal study and research. A professional portfolio is a collection of individual material, providing proof of personal growth, continuing professional development, lifelong learning and competence. A profile is a public version of the portfolio that summarises the content of the professional portfolio and can be submitted to professional bodies as proof of continuing professional development, or be used within an application for a position (Pearce, 2003).

All nurses and midwives on the professional register need to maintain a personal professional profile (Nursing and Midwifery Council, 2004c).

If a nurse or midwife wants to retain registration they have to provide evidence within their personal professional profile that they have spent at least five days (35 hours) within the previous three years updating their knowledge and skills (NMC, PREP Standard, Revised 2004c). Practitioners also need to have completed a minimum of 60 days (450 hours) of practice during the last 3 years to renew their registration.

The NMC calls it a personal professional profile and states that it is a record of career progress and professional development. The Health Professions Council (HPC) calls it a written portfolio and uses it to demonstrate CPD and lifelong learning. The HPC (2004) states that a portfolio:

- is a resource (that can be a hard copy or electronic format) that helps professionals to record, evaluate and reflect on their learning
- provides a tool for identifying ongoing learning needs and planning activity to meet these needs
- can be used to support a range of purposes (including preparation for annual appraisals, applying for a new job and seeking academic credit for work-based learning).

The HPC also links renewal of registration with evidence of continuing professional development, and its revised CPD rules have been implemented (Health Professions Council, 2005). Health care professionals are open to auditing of their portfolios from 2008 onwards. The HPC does not specify and monitor the number of hours of each registrant or number of study sessions attended, as there is a wish to be flexible to encompass the differing professional groups. Registrants are required to maintain a record of CPD activity and to make a self-declaration of their compliance to CPD standards. The Governing Council can ask at any time for a registrant to submit their CPD summary of recent work and practice as a profile. A pro forma is provided for the profile, and documentary evidence to support this needs to be available if required.

An effective portfolio is a visual representation of a practitioner's experience, strengths, abilities and skills. Cross-referencing, editing and imaginative paper management are important competencies in portfolio compilation. Recently, there has been general movement in portfolio development towards electronic portfolios, as these make use of current technology and can also allow for more creative and flexible visual records (Barrett, 2002).

Over to you

Review your portfolio of practice.

- Is it in an easily understandable format for someone to read?
- Does it present an accurate picture of your current level of practice?
- What do your reflections cover? (Reflections should not all be on issues of concern but rather offer a more balanced evaluation of the individual practitioner's abilities and potential.)
- Does your portfolio include evaluations of successful development to date?
- Identify what you could add or need to do to improve your portfolio.

Guidance on the structure/development of a CPD portfolio

Starting to develop a professional portfolio is often the most difficult part. Your portfolio should contain key documents such as your curriculum vitae (see template in Figure 8.2), current job description, person specification and your PDP. You should also include copies of certificates, records of learning activities, and academic awards. Whatever form your evidence takes, consider how it can be verified as your own work. For items where your authorship is not obvious, for example, a practice policy, you should try to obtain a verifying signature from an appropriate person, such as your line manager or clinical supervisor. Where you are using evidence from a joint project, you should detail which parts are specifically your work/actions. In many cases, evidence is paper-based and stored in a folder and will grow over time, so from the start keep a record of what is included, using an index to indicate where material is located in the folder. It is useful if you can triangulate your practice evidence, drawing on evidence that shows all aspects of professional practice (i.e. experience, reflection and theory). If you use evidence of patient care delivery make sure that patient confidentiality is maintained at all times.

Whatever format you choose, you need to split the evidence into logical sections, and if you are relating your evidence to a set of competences (Knowledge and Skills profile) it may be useful to use a cross-referencing grid or matrix. You need to get used to spotting possible sources of evidence. At first this will require you to gather a 'backlog' of evidence about your current practice. Once you have located this evidence you will only need to 'housekeep' the portfolio regularly, adding pieces of evidence to display new learning, for instance, completing a record of a learning event.

Name

Address

Telephone

E-mail

Profile
(Brief outline/like an advert summarising your key assets, as in the example below)

A nurse with six years' experience in surgery who is able to communicate effectively within a NHS organisation. Has a record of leading clinical teams and developing and implementing care pathways. High patient standards for care delivery are seen as a priority. Thrives on challenges, both inside and outside the ward setting, and is able to handle difficult clinical situations ensuring successful outcomes.

Personal details

Date of birth

Nationality

Other information e.g. Full, clean driving licence

Career history

Current post:

Previous positions.
(Include dates and main responsibilities).

Achievements e.g.
• Successfully implemented primary care on an acute surgical ward with 25 patients.
• Evaluated introduction of primary care by administering questionnaires to all staff within the multidisciplinary team.
• Designed and produced an introductory booklet for new members of staff and students; this has been well received on the ward and a similar format is being produced by other wards within the Trust.

Education and qualifications

Qualification, Institute, Dates undertaken.

Professional development

Courses attended, Dates undertaken.

Presentations at conferences

Figure 8.2 CV template

Record of learning activity

I am submitting evidence of learning from attending a study day into my portfolio as it demonstrates. . .

Study event/Nature of the learning activity
Date:
Title:
Briefly describe the learning activity (how many hours).

Describe what the learning activity consisted of: e.g. why you undertook this, what you did, what you expected to gain from this.

Outcome of the learning activity:
How did the learning relate to your work? Give evidence of learning

Give your personal view of how the learning could/has informed or influenced your work.

Do you have any plans for any follow-up learning?

What follows is one suggested structure for your portfolio, but there are many possible frameworks and the intention is not to limit you to this one. You will probably find it easier to create a structure from the start and add your material to the relevant section, rather than just adding material into one large file. Creating sections also means that your portfolio will be easier to reference or index and will be simpler for an assessor/reader to follow.

Example: Possible CPD portfolio structure

Section 1: Personal details

Name, Place of work, Line Manager, Mentor/Clinical Supervisor
Outline the work of your department and your current role.
CV
Job description
Job Specification
Knowledge and skills profile

Section 2: CPD and personal development plan

Individual objectives /PDP
Evidence of formal education
Work-based learning
Professional activities

Section 3: Professional practice

(a) Developing professional and ethical practice
(b) Developing client care
(c) Developing management and clinical leadership
(d) Developing as a lifelong learner

This chapter has provided you with an overview of assessment and the forms of evidence that can be used within portfolios. The movement from novice to expert practice has also been explored.

RRRRRRapid recap

Check your progress so far by working through each of the following questions.

1. What are the key differences between:
   a) formative and summative assessment of practice
   b) criterion-referenced and norm-referenced assessment of practice?
2. What are the level identifiers within Steinaker and Bell's (1979) experiential taxonomy?
3. Identify at least six forms of evidence that could be included within a practice portfolio.
4. What are the five levels that Benner (1984) identified regarding the development of nursing expertise?
5. What should be done about patient information, when placing evidence that links to patient care practice into an assessment-of-practice document?

If you have difficulty with one of these questions, read through the section again to refresh your understanding before moving on.

9 Managing constraints to learning through practice

Learning outcomes

By the end of this chapter you should be able to:

★ Understand how issues, such as high patient caseloads and service improvement initiatives, can have an impact on learning through practice

★ Appreciate how multidisciplinary working can facilitate or hinder learning through practice

★ Acknowledge the role of emotional labour within health care

★ Recognise effective strategies to minimise the effect of constraints within varying contexts of practice.

Introduction

Everyday work in clinical settings has, understandably, patient care as the priority and this can be viewed as constraining learning through practice. Busy workloads and the emotional content of health care delivery can create stress, when combined with providing support for learners. This chapter explores possible barriers to work-based learning, such as high patient caseloads, professional agendas, **emotional labour** and variations within different clinical settings. Ways to manage these constraints to learning through practice are discussed. Personal barriers to an individual's learning through practice, such as diminished self-confidence, being defensive to feedback and being uncomfortable with self-evaluation, have been explored in Chapter 5, so are not discussed in any depth here. Many factors can hinder or facilitate learning; some of these factors are identified in Figure 9.1.

Resource issues

Staff shortages can hamper learning, as existing staff need to manage high workloads and there is an increased reliance on temporary staff. Changes, such as those described in *Improving Working Lives* (DoH, 2000b) encourage flexible working and a work–life balance, but increase difficulties for senior nurses having to cover 24-hour care requirements and can make it difficult to roster students and their mentors together. With part-time working on the increase, a single student may work with a number of registered practitioners during their placement. Recruitment and retention is important as the loss of experienced nurses affects the continuity of care and the overall learning environment in the clinical area (Spouse, 2001). Also, shortages of placement opportunities in certain specialities can be compounded by the lack of adequately prepared clinical educators. Taking the time to meet with a clinical supervisor has benefits, and if staff are 'working flat out' this has a potentially detrimental effect on professional development.

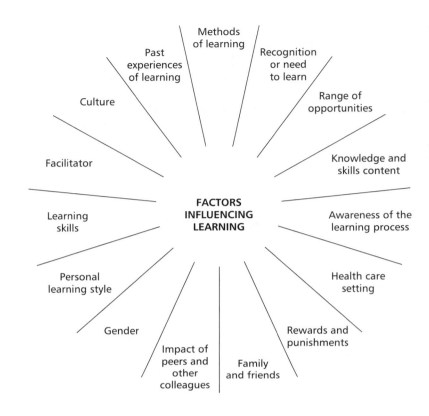

Keywords

Emotional labour

Emotional work is the actions an individual undertakes to manage their feelings when there is a gap between what they actually feel, and what they think they should feel. The term emotional labour indicates the emotional work done as part of a job and is governed by 'feeling rules' set by the employer. These unarticulated rules of social interactions indicate how deeply we should feel and for how long. Expectations for emotional labour tend to be linked to female-dominated work roles

Figure 9.1 Factors influencing learning (adapted from Connexions (2003) Learning and Young People. Department for Education and Skills, p. 12).

Reflective activity

Think about the following options for addressing the resources problems identified. What are the possible advantages and disadvantages of each of these solutions?

- Increasing the number of placements within the community (including the private sector).
- Using educators to support students or staff who are not from the same health care professional background (e.g. a student nurse spends time with a physiotherapist or ward clerk).
- Providing incentives or rewards for areas that offer a high level of support for student placement learning.
- Maximising the use of the working week for student allocations.
- Creating a cross-organisation educator role to support students.
- Developing interprofessional placements within specialities.

Circumstances affect learning, because of the opportunities offered (or withheld) by the context. It is more difficult to think flexibly during times of tension and stress so it is understandable that nurses and other health care professionals often act, think and behave in their 'usual' way even though this may not fit the situation (McAllister, 2003). Available evidence, the level of complexity and the practitioner's capabilities and disposition are factors that link with context to affect thinking. The time available and the complexity of the situation are important variables, and shortages of time force people to adopt a more intuitive approach, and intuitive routines help experienced staff to do things more quickly (Eraut, 2000b). Although routines vary between different clinical settings, the situated learning of these routines and the ability to perform accepted practice fluently within a setting is important to membership of a clinical team (Wigens, 2004).

👉 *Over to you*

Here is an example of a morning routine within one medical ward:

07.00 Handover from night shift to both teams. All patients are to have their observations and other charts reviewed and updated.

07.20 Handover is completed and drugs round commenced. Assist some patients who wish to meet washing and hygiene requirements prior to breakfast. Prepare patients for breakfast.

08.00 Serve breakfasts, giving assistance to those who require it. Document any food diaries and fluid charts. Once protected food time is complete, continue to assist other patients with hygiene needs. Ensure care is documented.

09.00 Day-specific commitments are commenced, e.g. preparation of patients for discharge, ward rounds.

10.00 Record any observations.

10.30 Staff breaks commence.

11.45 All staff should have returned from break.

11.45 Record any blood sugar measurements required.

12.00 Any patients with confirmed discharges should have departed; the reasons for any delays should be documented. Prepare patients for lunch (protected mealtime).

How useful do you think this ward routine would be to staff and students within this area. Find out about any routine within your current area of practice. Is this documented or simply in the heads of the staff in the area?

Professionals may be reluctant to talk about routines if they feel that these differ from those espoused in theories (such as individualised care) as they think that doing so will highlight inadequacies. Time pressure and uncertainty induce changes in the cognitive strategies used, influencing both the process and quality of decisions. Among the coping strategies utilised in situations of uncertainty are the use of planning schedules, and the synchronisation of tasks (McGrath and Rotchford, 1983). Uncertainty can be defined as the variability, degree of complexity, or novelty of a particular situation, and is linked to the character of the information available. Those who feel in control of their environment perceive uncertainty as a challenge, rather than as a threat, and are more likely to respond to this, using problem-solving strategies (Schuler and Jackson, 1986).

There are a number of strategies for coping with time pressure and information overload, including speeding up (acceleration), selecting the input of information (filtering), prioritising, using 'decision rules', omitting or avoiding, and locking on to one approach. When stress is high a decision is likely to be made based on what has previously been successful, and this decision may not be based on knowledge of all the available alternatives.

Learning to cope with (or even override) stress is part of 'situated learning' (Wigens, 2004). Nurses learn to assess, sort, and reshuffle the prioritisation of patients in their care. This prioritisation often uses a guiding framework, such as focusing on the 'sickest' patients and putting off aspects of care (such as support and advice giving) until later. By reviewing what has been provided, and looking back on past experiences, this guiding framework is evaluated for trustworthiness. Being able to constantly prioritise at speed and handle uncertainty whilst appearing calm and in control of the situation is the sign of an experienced nurse and something to which new staff nurses aspire.

Reflective activity

Think about the prioritisation frameworks used in your current area of work? Have they been made explicit? Could you outline them to a colleague?

Nurses within one case site were often found working at speed, and being 'busy' was signified to patients and other health care professionals by constant movement and a time-restricted approach to care interventions (Wigens, 2004). In this way, the resource constraints on nursing practice were made 'visible to the outside world' (Wenger, 1998; Wigens, 2004). Working at speed can leave time for emergencies that cannot be predicted. Eraut (1994) advocates that professions should openly discuss rationing and resource problems affecting care delivery, and I found that nurses in one case site talked freely of the perceived inadequacies such as available beds, caseloads, and their staffing establishments (Wigens, 2004). Being able to voice concerns regarding resource constraints does not, however, stop some nurses feeling frustrated with their perceived inability to control their work practices and workload (Wigens, 2004). Espoused theories of quality care involve giving care that is less rushed and is provided in a calm and controlled manner.

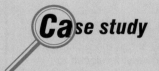

Case study research evidence

Wigens, L. (2004) A case study of registered (care of the adult) nurses' management of individual caring in multiple demands settings, and the influence on this of situated learning. Unpublished PhD thesis. University of East Anglia, Norwich.

This is a case study exploring the experiences of 22 nurses working within district, accident and emergency, medical, surgical, day surgery and care of the elderly care settings. Data was collected through career biography, critical incident analysis, interviewing and participant observation. Context-sensitive learning in relation to managing nursing care was examined. This study suggests a need to extend the notion of learning as a socially based activity occurring entirely in communities of practice (Lave and Wenger, 1991). The findings here indicate that much practical learning occurs when there is a dialogic relationship between a nurse's (professional and personal) identity and the nursing team (community of practice) in which he/she works. The research also found that because a considerable amount of 'knowing' in nursing is situated in participation in communities of practice, there is much to be gained from identifying frameworks that foster dialogue in those communities. The research concludes that there is considerable benefit to be had from the establishment of a 'facilitating culture' which enables situated leadership, particularly where such a culture addresses the fact that nursing practice is constrained by resource deficits and inequalities of power.

Paton (2003) found that practice educators are frequently thrown into situations that interrupt smooth clinical action and that they have to pause to make sense of what is going on, before they tackle the situation. This process is what novices witness when working with their practice educators, but they may not be able to understand unless they discuss and learn how individuals maintain personal boundaries and handle stress, thereby sustaining self (Paton, 2003). Nurses' perception is that they are expected to 'give of their own time' and that they are admired by others for doing so (Wigens, 2004). This expectation does, however, create problems for those who had previously worked in this way, when changing home commitments make it less realistic.

Changes in skill mix that increase the level of non-registered staff may also affect learning through practice. Skill mix involves professionals being willing to accept a form of interprofessional working that recognises the possibility that some needs may be met more effectively by lesser-trained staff. Skill mix can be achieved through delegation, substitution or diversification. However, there can be ambivalence within a nursing team about the role of support staff. Nurses value the contribution of assistants, but whether nurses accept this group as part of the nursing family is still open to debate (RCN, 2003).

Clinical Caseload . . .

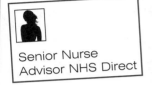

Senior Nurse Advisor NHS Direct

Nurses need to delegate care delivery to assistants safely and in line with training. Saunders (1998) suggests a framework of questions (originally developed for physiotherapists). If the answers to the questions are yes, the delegation should be safe, but it remains the responsibility of the qualified nurse to provide supervision for the health care assistant.

1 Is decision-making involved?

2 Is the task carried out frequently?

3 Does the patient require feedback following the task?

4 Is the response to treatment immediate?

5 Are the consequences of error not serious?

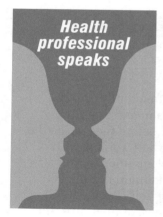

Health professional speaks

Staff nurse

I have to sit down for a good hour to get the care plans sorted, and it is difficult to make sure that everybody has had their care properly. Our care assistants now do so much of the care. We spend time in assessing their NVQ units that are about giving care. It is easy to get stuck into management role and actually only do the care plans, the pills, the doctors' rounds and not actually ever wash a patient. Which isn't right, really. Sometimes you don't have a choice and that can be quite upsetting. You know that you just can't be everywhere and you can only do so much, so it's better to support the learning of junior staff.

Interactions between health care professionals, nurses and support staff continue to be affected by the hierarchical structure that operates within clinical settings. Status can be a potential barrier to collegiate decision-making. Whatever the resource problem, it is necessary to remember that 'learning entails giving up old perceptions, comfortable assumptions and states of knowledge or ignorance and draws into question the past approaches, habits and mind-sets of individuals and groups' (Lines and Ricketts, 1994, p.165).

Specialities

The different cultures in clinical placements and specialities have been identified by students as having an impact on their learning (Pearcey and Elliott, 2004). Health care students have to learn to adapt to each placement, its characteristics and associated reputations by getting to know staff, and this is helped by having placements of a reasonable length (Crawford and Kiger, 1998).

Students have been found to go through three phases whilst on placement:

1   adaptation (becoming part of the community)

2   stabilisation (increased knowledge and skills)

3   consolidation (requiring reduced supervision) (Crawford and Kiger, 1998).

Reflective activity

What would be the optimum length of placement for a second-year student coming to the area you are presently in? How long (on average) does it take for you to adapt to a new clinical speciality? Have you found any particular area difficult to adapt to, and if so why do you think this was?

Pearcey and Elliott (2004) found some negative attitudes towards longer-stay patients. A fast turnover can limit the amount of time that nurses have to get to know the patients. In Melia's (1987) seminal study, students suggested that 'real nursing' occurred mostly on wards, happened at speed, and involved technical procedures or drug administration. Work described as 'proper nursing' focused on care of younger clients, was done at a fast pace, and feelings of success were measured in cure or discharge (Melia, 1987). It was not just regarded as 'passing the time' as in care of the elderly (Melia, 1987, p. 133). Melia (1987) suggests that students took the speciality as a reference point for the value of their own work and their preferences might simply reflect their stage of development as adults and nurses.

Smith's (1992) study also supported the increased prestige attached to technical and mental work. Students were affected by the atmosphere of the clinical area, particularly if nurses were viewed as not making the effort to talk with their patients and build up the nurse–patient relationship (Pearcey and Elliott, 2004). By contrast, when a clinical area had high morale, a positive atmosphere and encouraged staff development, the students were motivated in their continued interest in nursing. The students within Pearcey and Elliott's (2004) study were concerned that so much of their learning through practice came from negative experiences and that, through a need to 'fit in', they too could become socialised into a less caring approach to patients.

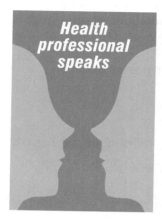

Charge nurse working in an Intensive Care Unit

I have thought about what can reduce stress for students and I try to reduce the chances of this. Intensive care can be a frightening environment for anyone coming into it for the first time. I try to make my expectations of the student clear and achievable, and I give regular feedback. To help reduce their anxiety, I share any concerns about their care delivery away from the patient and relatives. I feel that it is very important that students are equitably treated, so whatever their own past experiences I make sure that they are immersed slowly into taking on a clinical workload.

Emotional labour

You may, perhaps, take the view that emotions just happen to you and that you are not fully responsible for them; however, they involve a degree of cognition and are also 'socioculturally constituted'. A clinical team's belief systems and values affect the capacity and characteristics of emotional expression. Hochschild (1983), who suggests that 'feeling rules' are socially variable and historically changing, has focused on uncomfortable emotion management within work settings. Staff within clinical settings do find time for 'fun' and humour as this can help them to confront the less enjoyable aspects of practice, develop camaraderie and a sense of community (Castro *et al.*, 1999). Emotional labour required for caring for people in distress is often balanced by emotional release through humour and jokes (Wigens, 2004). Maeve (1998) found that the humorous issues and content of jokes could be considered shocking or inappropriate, if heard by people outside a clinical setting.

Reflective activity

Have you noticed the use of humour within clinical settings to relieve stress? Did this ever concern you, or appear 'inappropriate' when you were on clinical placement or in a new locality?

In the past, nurses were encouraged to appear busy and were advised to maintain a professional barrier to avoid becoming emotionally involved with patients (Menzies, 1960). Concentrating on 'tasks' can detach nurses from feelings and reduce the nurse–patient relationship. Menzies (1960) suggested that social structures within nursing, such as the routines of care were a form of defence, to avoid anxiety, guilt, doubts and uncertainty, by denying the significance of the individual. Menzies suggested that it was perhaps the most defensive individuals who stay in nursing and that those unable to cope with the rigidity of the system, the elimination of personal discretion and growth left the profession.

Parsons' (1968) seminal work identified that professional socialisation creates affect-neutral practitioners who avoid emotional involvement with clients. James (1992) suggested that in practice individualised care may only amount to finding out enough about patients to know when to interrupt routines to attend to individual requirements. Allen (2000) found that although nurses wanted to involve family and friends in care, implementing this in practice placed additional demands on their limited time. When the management of nursing care results in a requirement to speed-up 'the human assembly line', this makes 'genuine' personal service harder to deliver and it becomes virtually impossible to deliver emotional labour and individualised psychological care (Wigens, 1997).

The claim that there has been movement from the domination of physical care and limited nurse–patient communication to more holistic care is still open to challenge by studies that report similar superficial, task-focused communication (Hewinson, 1999). A number of models (types) of nurse–patient relationships have been identified:

Models of practitioner–patient relationships

1 Nurse centred

This emphasised the patient's dependence on the health carer. Care giving was determined by the nurse who was viewed as more 'knowledgeable' than the patient. Care is delivered in the patient's best interest.

2 Technical relationship

Nursing is seen as a clinical science, where skilled technical, objective care is competently delivered without imposing any of the carer's values or wishes. The patient may have the ultimate responsibility for determining needs, but the nurse informs and has current evidence and skills to impart.

3 Patient centred

The nurse works alongside the patient, negotiating the role of the nurse as applicable to the situation and individual patient needs. Within this model, there is the possibility for the nurse and patient to 'know' each other as people.

4 Therapeutic relationship

Therapeutic relationship requires the nurse to respect and have genuine interest in the person, to show emotional warmth, tolerance and non-judgemental acceptance of the patient. It also calls for the practitioner to use 'self' in nursing interactions, whilst maintaining awareness of their limitations and adherence to ethical codes. The patient plays a part in a therapeutic relationship by trusting and co-operating with the intervention and being motivated to understand the treatment/ care.

Reflective activity

During your time working in various clinical settings have you seen all of these forms of the nurse–patient relationship? Do you think that patient problems, the length of the patient episode or the age of the patient influenced the nurse–patient relationships observed?

Perhaps you identified during the reflective activity that not every patient requires a deep practitioner–patient relationship, but that wherever possible it should be patient centred. Eraut (1994) suggests that there is a close link between client centredness and continuing to develop one's professional knowledge. As nurses and other health care practitioners have started to research and explore the nurse–patient relationship, there has been increasing interest in the concept of emotional labour.

From an emotional labour approach, emotions are brought in line with feeling rules by two means:

- Surface acting – in this case, the nurse puts on the expressive visage or body stance of the emotion in the hope of stimulating the authentic feeling, changing feeling from the outside in.

- Deep acting – here, more profound strategies, such as imaging and verbal and physical prompting are used, modifying bodily or mental states, changing the feeling from the inside out (Hochschild, 1983). An example of prompts to deep acting might be the way the nurses talk to each other during a handover when they are discussing the care of a dying patient and his or her relatives.

Student nurses have been found to experience anxiety and stress because their emotional labour was largely unrecognised and undervalued, and their workloads meant that there was only time to meet the physical and technical needs of patients (Smith, 1992). The 'little things' of caring were not being recognised or costed in the work environment that emphasised 'getting the work done' and rewarded non-patient-oriented activities (Smith, 1992). The concept of emotional labour helps in understanding how emotions have become a commodity in the work environment, just like technical skills, such as prescribing.

Overt examples of lack of caring from senior nursing staff can affect the future working of junior staff, so role models for care giving and emotional labour are important for student nurses.

> ## Reflective activity
>
> With another person, reflect on an incident where you observed an experienced nurse acting as a role model for psychological care giving. What did you particularly notice about their practice?
>
> How did it feel to discuss and share this incident with another person? Reflective learning itself can be seen as a form of emotional labour, as nurses share and work through difficult issues and problems with other nurses.

Nurses working with more insight into the home situation and usual lifestyle of the patient feel that this helps develop patient–nurse relationships. 'Having a picture' of the patient as a person in the world is personal knowledge that affected care delivery (Wigens, 2004). Perhaps this is part of the 'imaging' that Hochschild (1983) suggests is required for 'deep acting'. The length of time and continuity of patient care is seen as a contributory factor in allowing deeper, therapeutic relationships to develop (Wigens, 2004).

Senior nurses within a clinical setting play a crucial role in developing the social construction of emotional work, setting the 'tone' for staff, patients and visitors (Wilson-Barnett *et al.*, 1995). Senior nurses need to be open to new ideas, allow a flexible approach to routines and be supportive to staff so that individualised care can be provided (James, 1992). Lawler (1991) found that 'expert nurses' achieved a fine balance between showing concern and care for the patient whilst also appearing professional. During a working day, various situations require differing degrees of emotional work, and this can range from a minimal level, when giving routine 'basic' care, to a greater level, when caring for a dying patient (Bolton, 2001). Bolton (2001) stresses the emotional complexity within nursing work by employing the term 'emotional jugglers' to highlight nurses' capacity to present a variety of faces. Mentors and 'link lecturers' assume a key role for students in learning about emotional work.

When Priest (1999) compared 'expert' and 'novice' understanding of psychological care, she identified that experts considered information giving as a major aspect, whereas novices placed more emphasis upon personal qualities. Experts concentrated on handling emotions and novices focused on facilitating the expression of emotions; Priest (1999) suggested that this is because experts are more mindful that encouraging patients to 'open up' may require time which is unavailable owing to competing demands and priorities. According to Priest (1999), the specific training programmes in psychological care have not been adopted by nurses, as there is some doubt as to whether psychological care can be taught, whether it is solely developed through experience or indeed whether all nurses can develop psychological care-giving abilities. The nurses' own life experiences are seen as integral to their patient care.

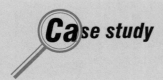

Emotional labour and patient expectations

A team meeting was being held – lead by a senior nurse for the unit – as there had been some complaints regarding the lack of 'caring attitudes' displayed by the nursing staff towards some patients. The group was split into two smaller discussion groups and the following issues were raised and discussed.

Some nurses said that their critical reflections on practice involved reviewing how much 'feeling' they had integrated into their care giving and that the workload on the ward had reduced the level of this from what they would like to have delivered. Others said that not getting 'too involved' was important and that this formed part of their personal philosophy of care. Both groups agreed that professional working required a balance of personal value judgements about how much time to spend with individual patients. One nurse was seen as a role model for caring skills within the ward team, even though she was not one of the most experienced members of staff. She talked about the need to 'give something' of herself as an open and honest 'real person', to build effective patient relationships, but did not feel that this was realistic for all patients within their care.

The ward nurses talked about bringing their personal learning from their home life to their nursing and vice versa. Nurses' personal knowledge from their home life meant that they accepted that they 'made contact' with certain patients only, and with others they were only likely to develop superficial relationships. There was a process of selecting the depth of involvement with individual patients, which related to the priorities within the clinical area at the time. There was consensus that emotional involvement with a patient and relatives was demanding but can also make a role feel more worthwhile. The staff had been very upset about the complaints about their caring communications.

What suggestions do you think could help these ward staff work on this aspect of their practice? How might they manage their caring and emotional labour to meet their patients' expectations?

Students learn to 'tune into' the emerging priorities within a placement and to calls for situated understanding of the emotional labour requirements. Student nurses accumulated knowledge of emotional labour through experience and were able to talk reflectively about nursing experience with staff and colleagues. Most nurses expect their psychological care and empathy to develop through trial-and-error learning, the passage and exposure of practice, observation of role models and feedback from patients, with reflective diaries or portfolios assisting this process (Priest, 1999).

Increasing nursing experience does not necessarily equate with improved communication and psychological caring (Wigens, 2004). The circumstances when nurses are more likely to become 'personally close' with patients include when patients are critically or acutely ill, suffering psychological distress, dying, angry and aggressive, or when the patient or situation closely mirrors people or situations from the nurses' personal lives (Wigens, 2004). It can prove difficult for students to observe 'emotionally challenging situations' as an observational role may affect the dynamics of a difficult clinical situation. This aspect of practice, therefore, has become something that junior nurses learn through observation of fragments of patient and relative interactions, and discussions with experienced staff, but mainly through doing.

The constant requirement to undertake emotional labour can affect the meaning that nurses attach to their own personal problems, as they compare their own issues to those of patients within their care, and this meant that they viewed them from a different perspective (Wigens, 2004). Interactions (formal and informal, social and professional contact during work hours) between nurses and colleagues are viewed as important to supporting caring, and nurses generally indicate a high level of satisfaction with these. Informal support networks often comprise other nurses who play a crucial role in maintaining stability by making themselves available to discuss a distressing clinical situation (Wigens, 2004). In order to make professional judgements in an emotionally charged situation, nurses learn to vent their personal feelings later, after the event (Wigens, 2004). A sign of nursing maturity was that, even though 'some part of a difficult incident' remains with the nurse, they avoid bringing this home (Wigens, 2004). Nurses use their emotions on a daily basis in their practice, selecting the depth and level of their emotional work.

Service improvement

Modernisation of health services requires a breaking down of traditional barriers to find new and flexible ways of thinking and doing, calling for creative responses. Implicit within service improvement is the ability to change, develop new roles, interprofessional working, lifelong learning and collegiate working (Gough, 2001). Service improvement can place additional demands on nurses, requiring them to implement change, often to meet government targets, whilst still having to complete the ongoing clinical care. Many health carers are sceptical about the finance available for properly supporting modernisation and there is a perception that managers are more concerned with finance than they are with patient care (Callaghan, 2003; Wigens, 2004).

The changes required to implement evidence-based practice can sometimes tip the fine balance of everyday coping, where much of this practice is based on tacit knowledge, sometimes made explicit through reflection. Change, even when acknowledged as improving patient care, can overload and stretch clinical staff who have 'learnt to manage'. Modernisation within nursing has lead to the ownership and co-ordination of patient flow, and patient flow can become the management of people into bed spaces rather than seeing patients as individuals. Nursing teams adapt their working to help 'meet a target', implement evidence-based change (Heitlinger, 1999) and empower patients, in such a way that change is minimised (Wigens, 2004).

Clinical teams who feel a sense of 'change overload' more easily accept change if patient care is improved as an outcome. The overall success of a change can also be dependent on whether nurses feel that the nursing team has ownership of the change. Colleagues are easily accessible and able to adapt messages to counter individual, organisational and environmental barriers and are able to harness multiple approaches to changing practice, including one-to-one educational approaches, influencing clinical audit agendas, clinical teaching, mentorship and role modelling.

Over to you

Find out about the service improvement structure within your organisation. What initiatives are in place to help meet the 10 high-impact changes? For further national information on this, go to the following website and search for the latest modernisation initiatives: www.dh.gov.uk

Modernisation has lead to the development of expanded roles and the re-engineering of nursing roles, (Tye and Ross, 2000). Service improvements can be a route for career diversity for nurses and other health care professions, such as specialist, advanced practitioner and consultant roles that add to the highly differentiated careers. New roles increase opportunities for retaining and developing senior nurses, raising the profile of the profession, without the overall caring motivations being lost (Callaghan, 2003). Opposition to the medicalisation of nurses' role and identity and to potential de-skilling competes alongside the increased professional and career opportunities (Tye and Ross, 2000). Perceived inequities in workload between general and specialist staff can occur along with a blurring of the distinct or unique differences between nursing and medicine. New roles within nursing inevitably create uncertainty owing to the reconstructing of professional identity (Williams and Sibbald, 1999). Nurse practitioners and specialist nurses can feel a sense of isolation from the rest of the nursing staff, made tangible through different uniforms and different geographical locations (Tye and Ross, 2000). Foucault (1972) believed that it is through discourse that the social production of meaning occurs and that power and knowledge are inextricably linked. Specialisation has probably gained power and legitimacy from its knowledge base; however, by the very process of differentiation and the establishment and maintenance of distinct identities, it can lead to reduced collaboration and to tribalism.

> ### *Over to you*
>
> Find out about the specialist nurse and nurse practitioner roles that visit or link with your current clinical area. Take opportunities to learn through practice by shadowing one of these staff for a shift or during a patient interaction. Discuss their role and what knowledge underpins their practice.

⌐ₙ *Keywords*

Hegemony

Hegemony is an organising principle or common-sense ideology that permeates throughout society and is socialised into everyday life and accepted by the majority

Armstrong and Armstrong (1996) argue that there is a growing fragmentation of nursing work due to the **hegemony** of the medical model, with tasks being reassigned to different categories of nurses.

Tasks that might have been incorporated into nursing have been moved out, for example, administration and food delivery (Heitlinger, 1999). There is already a division of labour in nursing teams through the separation of the assessment and technical care, done by registered nurses, from the 'basic' patient care that is commonly undertaken by support staff. This can create a sense of tension that what is mainly a support worker role contrasts with the symbolic 'hands on' role that has previously been regarded as 'real nursing'. There has been dissociation between the conception and execution of much nursing work as registered nurses take on more of the 'clean' work, such as discharge planning (Lawler, 1991; Wigens, 2004). This separation of nursing decision-making from care delivery is underpinned by the view that 'mental work' has a higher status in comparison with 'manual work' (Wigens, 1997). Armstrong and Armstrong (1996) talk of the growing fragmentation of nursing work through this division of labour, making communication and learning even more important for all members of a nursing team.

Increased standardisation and the use of information technology means that some nurses perceive that the requirement for professional judgement and autonomy has been reduced, and inflexible barriers are being created (Wigens, 2004). However, the introduction of new technology can also create an opportunity for learning. New technologies are more accepted if they have a direct impact on workload, but the initial time taken to learn about new equipment must 'pay back' quickly through improved patient care in order for a clinical team to continue investing time in training (Wigens, 2004).

Evidence base

Have a look at some of the information on these websites:

● www.nhsdirect.nhs.uk

● www.connectingforhealth.nhs.uk

How have technology and the increased access to information influenced learning through practice?

Student nurses have been found to have a deficit in their knowledge of how to effectively improve clinical practice involving the management of change, even though this should be embedded in all health care professional training. Reflection mainly takes a written form submitted to a lecturer, and students want to be given feedback on their reflection whilst in the clinical setting (Kyrkjebø and Hage, 2005). There is a mismatch between what students learn about quality patient care and what they actually observe in practice. Kyrkjebø and Hage (2005), who used a focus group methodology with a sample of 27 Norwegian student nurses, suggest that there is a need to encourage reflection and openness to allow students to scrutinise why errors and omissions in care occur.

Improvement knowledge and processes can be separated into four elements:

● knowledge of the organisational system in which health care is delivered and of how involved patients are in making decisions about care

● knowledge of the variation in processes, products and people and how to measure this

● knowledge of accountability, psychology and social working and the approach to change

● knowledge of how to link theory to action so that the knowledge becomes locally useful (Batalden and Stoltz, 1993).

The development of improvement knowledge can be helped by learning the 'plan–do–study–act' (PDSA) cycle (Batalden and Stoltz, 1993) (See Figure 9.2).

The PDSA cycle gives a systematic way of developing new knowledge through learning by experience. However, some health professionals seem to lack the ability to see health care delivery as a process which can be identified, mapped, measured and studied for variation (Mohammed, 2004). An environment that harnesses the PDSA cycle and encourages thinking about 'working smarter' needs to be supported. Nursing can be viewed as 'doing', rather than also about talking and discussing. Time to discuss and plan service improvement changes should be balanced alongside 'doing' within clinical environments and is a crucial facet in learning through practice.

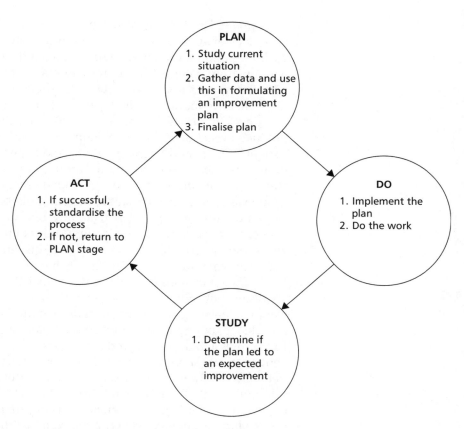

Figure 9.2 PDSA cycle (Batalden and Stoltz, 1993)

Interprofessional working

Nurses compare themselves with other health care professionals, and gender issues (as nursing continues to be a predominantly female-dominated occupation) still continue to influence interprofessional working (Witz, 1992). Nursing has devoted considerable attention to its status as a profession and its subsequent power basis in relation to doctors (Snelgrove and Hughes, 2000). Interprofessional working requires situated learning, and the way that nurses perceive their occupation plays a significant part in determining working relationships (Wigens, 1998).

Gender issues affect professionalisation. Professional projects are strategies of occupational closure that seek a monopoly over skills and competencies, and nursing is perceived to be adopting a dual-closure strategy (Witz, 1992), aiming to prevent other professions from controlling nursing and delegating their 'unwanted tasks' (Wigens, 1997). Nurses are viewed, in some of the literature, as in conflict and as an oppressed and marginalised group (Farrell, 2001). Complaints often cover lack of autonomy, even though nurses are responsible over the 24-hour period for patients in their care, and a perceived need to protect patients from potential harm from others, for example, doctors. Although nurses take responsibility for their own actions, they often work in a collective manner when trying to change another professional's practice (Ohlen and Segesten, 1998; Wigens, 2004). These socially produced vocabularies of complaint often focus on 'what is best for the patient' (Ohlen and Segesten, 1998) and allow nurses to reassert their unity with the wider occupational group. This culture within nursing has a direct impact on what is learnt through practice. To develop frameworks for practice that are meaningful, there needs to be movement towards open debate among all health care professionals concerning decisions. Strong communities of practice should be able to withstand disagreement and learn from this, and use other conflict-management strategies rather than avoidance (Wigens, 2004).

Professional 'boundary patrolling' is usually reinforced by highlighting an absence of codified knowledge in the group wishing to take on the work usually done by others, even though much of the specialist knowledge underpinning practice is actually situated and personal. Interprofessional working and learning is challenging, complex and controversial (Hammick, 1998). Interprofessional collaboration is often not achieved in practice, or seen as meaningful and effective for patients (Hammick, 1998). Wilson and Pirrie (2000) have found that opportunities for interprofessional working are more successful when new coalitions are formed between allied health professionals and nurses, as power issues are less historically based. The value placed on making regular contact with patients can affect nurses' perceptions of other health care professionals, meaning that the strongest alliances are with the staff who spend time on a regular basis with patients (Wigens, 2004).

Reflective activity

Take a look at what one nurse said about another professional group. Think about what she is suggesting and how this could be a barrier to interprofessional learning.

'The day-to-day hassles like social workers: I do appreciate that they have as many problems, but, when I have got a social worker who isn't putting in care fast enough so that I can discharge this person home, I get a bit. . .You get a consultant coming round saying, "Why hasn't this person gone home?" Then you're "piggy-in-the-middle". When we're stressed we tend to go into our own factions/corners, but to get things done you need to work together as your goal is ultimately the same.'

The style of normal interaction in the clinical setting is an important variable affecting interprofessional learning in practice. Case conferences and ward rounds are often the sites for encounters that underpin interprofessional working and involve a daily mixture of submission and assertion (Wigens, 2004). However, there can be a lack of forums for interprofessional discussion, such as case conferences, ward rounds or interprofessional team meetings, or the timing of these can affect nursing involvement. When nurses are not actively engaged in patient care decisions, they can perceive this as indicating that their contribution to patient care is not valued. Where interprofessional communication is promoted and supported, learning within the practice area is enhanced (Wigens, 2004). Situated learning between different health care professionals is highly valued, but unfortunately not frequently observed (Pirrie *et al.*, 1998; Wigens, 2004).

Over to you

Bruce (1980) suggests that the effectiveness of a team can be classified as nominal, convenient or committed. The classifications are:

- nominal team – there is only very limited teamwork occurring
- convenient team – a clinician (often the doctor) delegates work to other health care practitioners
- committed team – the team members invest time and energy into their teamwork.

Consider the multidisciplinary team (MDT) within which you are presently working; if you had to categorise it, which of Bruce's three terms would best describe the level of working?

How does this compare with other MDTs within which you have worked?

Nurses spend time on the development of sound working relationships with other professionals (Pirrie *et al.*, 1998). The nurses in one case site saw that working with less-experienced health care professionals at the start of their careers was a unique opportunity to make an impact on future interprofessional working (Wigens, 2004). They felt in a stronger position in relation to other health care professionals, if they were working in a speciality rather than in a more general setting, and were more likely to give advice in an open manner to other professionals (Wigens, 2004). Experienced staff may invest 'ring-fenced' time to focus on this leadership component of their role. Effective interprofessional working is helped by the development of communication channels and a team spirit across professions. Gradual development of interpersonal support that extends beyond the workplace contributes to a 'team feeling', and tends to surface when a clinical area has had to deal with an emotionally demanding situation.

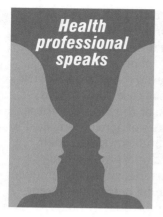

Sister (nurse) on a general surgical ward

We tend to have a very good relationship with the doctors, the consultants and the house officers. They're straight out of college and they tend to take our advice. I mean, it's all first-name terms and they support us and we support them you know . . . when they're in tears we comfort them and they do the same for us really. We definitely try and promote the multidisciplinary team; the nurse involvement probably depends on the consultant involved, and the ones we work with mainly treat us as professionals.

The strength of interprofessional relationships and working is related to the vigour of teamworking, networking and emotional labour (Wigens, 2004). Situated learning about other health care professionals involves not just an understanding of their role, but knowing them as 'authentic' people. If this has been achieved, it appears to reduce the stress related to interprofessional working and increase respect for each other's unique contribution to patient care (Wigens, 2004). Interprofessional teamworking needs committed 'champions' who share their vision and make working together a reality, using their networks and clinical practice experience (Pirrie *et al.*, 1998). By working together and learning clarity about each other's roles, practitioners may take up opportunities for interprofessional supervision, coaching, feedback and sharing insights (Wilson and Pirrie, 2000).

Interprofessional team working in clinical practice can strengthen learning through experience. Mutual respect is developed when students and qualified staff from a range of health care professions learn to work with each other and to participate collaboratively. The outcome is more effective and safer health care. Health care practitioners meet the increasingly complex demands placed on them by learning to cope from moment to moment in the clinical environment with limited resources. Structures to support situated learning should be flexible, allowing forms of tacit knowledge to be made more explicit as nurses learn to interact and improvise in ways that make sense to their community. These authentic learning environments reflect the way that knowledge is used and developed in 'real life', by encouraging multiple perspectives and changing roles for members of the community, providing support and the opportunity for members to reflect on their practice and the chance to make their learning explicit. The art in developing nursing is to foster rather than organise communities of practice and to find resources and connections without overwhelming nursing teams with organisational meddling. As well as the tangible effects on skill development, performance, decision-making and risk-taking, fostering communities of practice could also improve relationships, a sense of belonging and enquiry, and increase professional confidence and identity formation for members. This is discussed further in the final chapter.

RRRRR*Rapid recap*

Check your progress so far by working through each of the following questions.

1 What strategies may nurses use to cope with high workloads, time pressures and information overload?

2 What three phases do Crawford and Kiger (1998) suggest students progress through whilst on clinical placement?

3 Outline the main aspects of the four models of practitioner–patient relationship.

4 What is meant by the term 'emotional labour'?

5 What do the letters PDSA stand for in the service improvement cycle?

6 How might a multidisciplinary team that could be described as 'committed' (Bruce, 1980) show that they are working interprofessionally?

If you have difficulty with one of these questions, read through the section again to refresh your understanding before moving on.

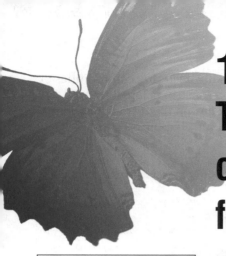

10
The wider context: creating an environment for learning

Learning outcomes

By the end of this chapter you should be able to:

★ Explain the main curricular changes that have occurred within health professional education

★ Appreciate the importance of fostering a learning culture at all levels of an organisation

★ Value the range of educational roles that support learning through practice

★ Understand how higher education institutes and service providers need to work together to optimise learning through practice.

Introduction

In this, the final, chapter we look at the wider context that supports learning through practice. You will gain an awareness of how the learning climate within a clinical setting is affected by changing curricula and policy implementation. Although much of the discussion looks at nursing, professional education within nursing mirrors that of many health care professions. The chapter explores key educational roles not based solely within clinical settings, including practice educators, link lecturers and professional and practice development roles, and stresses the importance of academic and service partnership working. This chapter brings together many of the themes that you encountered within previous chapters and that contribute to developing effective communities of practice within clinical placements.

Changing curricula

In nursing, there has been a movement away from what was broadly apprenticeship training with education delivered in NHS nursing departments to pre-registration programmes of education delivered within higher education institutes (HEIs) and leading to a minimum academic qualification at diploma level. There has also been increased access to post-registration qualifications at degree and higher degree levels.

Sometimes, an 'unfortunate split' between cognitive and practical skills has inadvertently been reinforced by a curriculum development team, with 'practical skills being relegated to a position of 'secondary importance' (Elkan and Robinson, 1993). Decontextualised skills learnt in school are not transferable to the workplace, and the fragmented, information-driven view of professional knowledge leads to a piecemeal collection of knowledge without an understanding of how it fits together (Bechtel *et al.*, 1999; Richardson, 1999). Edmond (2001) suggests that education for all practice disciplines is undergoing a paradigm shift, where the value of practical education and experience will be better understood and integrated with theoretical knowledge. This cultural shift requires a movement away from 'clinical education by default' (Edmond, 2001), reduced emphasis on front-loading theory, and increased structure for practical experiences (Eraut *et al.*, 1998).

Looking back on curricular changes within nursing, it is clear that a radical educational shift occurred with the implementation of 'Project 2000' pre-registration curricula. The major aim of Project 2000 curricula was to deliver knowledgeable nurses for the future. The key changes involved student nurses learning broad life sciences, health promotion, evidence-based practice, and common subject areas with other student nurses from four main branches (adult, child, learning disabilities and mental health nursing) early on in their careers (Slevin and Buckenham, 1992). This was achieved through supernumerary student status at diploma level. The curricular revolution that occurred was also mirrored in post-registration initiatives. Students expressed frustration at what they regarded as irrelevant subjects forming such a large component of the pre-registration curriculum, when they were more concerned with learning practical skills (Corlett, 2000). Students saw theory as decontextualised, making it difficult to apply in practice, and learning on placement was given more credence (Hislop *et al.*, 1996). An additional outcome from this curricular change was a reduction in nurse teacher contact with clinical settings (RCN, 2004).

In 1999, the Department of Health and the United Kingdom Central Council for Nursing, Midwifery and Health Visiting (UKCC) recommended the strengthening of education and training for nurses (UKCC/DoH, 1999). The 'fitness for practice' model called for increased flexibility within curricula, partnership working between HEIs and NHS Trusts, and initiatives to ensure that students were able to meet the future roles envisaged for registered nurses (DoH, 2000c).

Main changes in 'fitness for practice' curriculum

- Increased student intakes to meet NHS requirements which required additional practice placements
- Flexible approaches to access and accreditation of prior (experiential) learning (APEL)
- Earlier allocations of students to practical placements from the start of their course
- An identified 'base ward' to increase 'ownership' of the students by the service providers
- Improved integration of theory and practice throughout the course, with an emphasis on clinical practice and the development of transferable critical appraisal skills

continued

- Strengthened partnership links between higher education institutes and NHS Trusts
- A shorter common foundation programme (reduced from 18 months to 1 year)
- Wider assessment of practice skills by practice supervisors (mentors) through the development of practice evidence
- A need to demonstrate competence at the end of pre-registration education with a period of preceptorship following registration

Learning-centred curricula identify learning outcomes reflecting current nursing practice and the user's perspective (Bailey, 2005) and use authentic assessment to evidence these (Candela *et al.*, 2006). One method advocated for integrating theory and practice 'camps' is problem-based learning, which is increasingly in use (Bechtel *et al*, 1999). Problem-based learning involves the simultaneous addressing of skills, knowledge and professional attitudes through group work and experiential learning which may transfer more easily to the clinical context (Ramsden, 1992). Richardson (1999) also suggests that the use of more innovative teaching methods, such as practice videos or tape-recordings/transcripts of patient–professional and interprofessional health care interactions, as a way of reducing the theory–practice divide, could be debated in the academic setting.

Key points | *Top tips*

Teaching methods that support the integration of theory and practice are:

- Problem-based learning (can be based around one patient case, a patient problem, a clinical skill, an ethical or professional dilemma)
- Team teaching involving lecturers and clinical staff
- Accrediting work-based learning
- Recording and reviewing role-play communications
- Well-designed interactive e-learning with sufficient computer access time and skills (Atack and Rankin, 2002)
- Access to evidence-based information within academic and practical settings
- Clinical skills laboratories that allow the simulation of health care environments
- Action learning sets
- Patient teaching
- Tutorials and discussion groups
- Workshops
- Personal development plans

Evidence base

The involvement of patients in teaching health care professionals has most successfully been integrated into mental health and learning disabilities curricula. Take a look at the following two articles:

- McGarry, J. and Thorn, N. (2004) How users and carers view their involvement in nurse education. *Nursing Times*, **100**(18), 36–39.
- Costello, J. and Horne, M. (2001) Patients as teachers? An evaluative study of patients' involvement in classroom teaching. *Nurse Education in Practice*, **1**(2), 94–102.

Health professional education has undergone a number of changes over the past 20 years, reflecting national educational trends and service changes. Nursing practice is changing, with nurses in acute settings caring for increasingly complex patient problems and sicker patients, and nurses in primary care settings working with raised levels of chronic illness and encouraging self-care wherever possible (RCN, 2004). This trend is likely to lead to a shift from hospital-based care to community-based care (Wanless, 2004). These service changes create challenges for curricular planning, which needs to offer increased student participation in community-based experiences (Gaines *et al.*, 2005).

Health care curricula are now required to integrate interprofessional learning to prepare staff adequately for their future work roles (ENB/DoH, 2001). Interprofessional education incorporates the arrangements made for people from different disciplines and professions to learn with each other, and it has been suggested that the term 'interprofessional' implies that professions should learn from and about each other to improve collaboration, rather than just learn side by side (CAIPE, 1997). Advocates of interprofessional learning perceive that it promotes teamwork and cultivates collaborative practice. Interprofessional education involves the application of the principles of interactive adult learning (discussed in Chapter 2) to interprofessional group-based learning (Wigens, 1999).

Reflective activity

Think about when you have participated in interprofessional learning. What was the subject area? (Common areas for interprofessional learning often include communication, documentation, problem solving, critical thinking, management, research, ethics, reflective practice and clinical supervision.) In your opinion, was the topic an appropriate area for interprofessional learning and was it handled well, so that all participants' contributions were valued?

Opportunities for nurses and other health care professionals to learn together should be taken: not just by getting professionals into the classroom together but by sharing learning through meaningful projects. Being critically aware of the influence of context (or presage factors) can inform interprofessional education decisions (Freeth and Reeves, 2004). There are logistical difficulties in organising interprofessional educational curricula, and a clinical hierarchy can affect interprofessional working, with some members being perceived as having more professional knowledge and status (Pirrie *et al.*, 1998). Placing professionals together in multi-disciplinary groups does not necessarily guarantee the development of a shared understanding. For instance, student nurses who shared lectures with medical and allied health professional students in their first year did not appear to develop an enthusiastic approach to multidisciplinary working (Pirrie *et al.*, 1998). Student nurses often sat in segregated groups, and they expressed concerns about the lack of opportunities to consolidate their own sense of professional identity before introducing interprofessional education within their programme (Pirrie *et al.*, 1998).

Evidence as to the effectiveness of interprofessional education from the first systematic reviews indicates that interprofessional education is happening in a wide range of health care programmes at pre- and post-qualification levels (Barr *et al.*, 1999). Positive changes in knowledge and skills have been found, and some evidence shows that interprofessional learning has an impact on patient outcomes (Barr *et al.*, 1999; Hammick, 2000). It is suggested that health care professionals should be educated to function as team members, which would be helped by a consensus about the competences that graduates should achieve (Stephenson *et al.*, 2002).

Parity in educational curricula has become important, and the RCN (2004) suggests that the transition to an all graduate nursing profession has a certain inevitability, as most health care professions have their initial qualifications linked to gaining a degree. There has been, however, scepticism about advocating an all-graduate nursing workforce (Burke and Harris, 2000). Miers (2002) suggests that there is anti-intellectualism within nursing which has been fuelled by those in practice who critique nursing academia. This view is supported by the suggestion that there has been a denigration of practice by those who are solely based within nursing institutes of higher education, with these nursing academics valuing propositional knowledge over other forms of knowledge. Heitlinger (1999) suggests that the movement of nursing education into higher education has benefited nurses, as the location of their education within universities has increased their political position in comparison with other health care professionals. Those advocating a degree-level pre-registration qualification argue that theoretical learning does not preclude practical ability (RCN, 2004).

Nurse educational programmes are particularly appreciated if they assess 'learning in practice', thus allowing individuals to immerse themselves in practice (Wigens, 2004). Immersion in practice early on in a nursing career is seen as the way to learn nursing (UKCC, 1999). Qualified staff view students as needing a lengthy time in practice, greater than four weeks, and believe that supernumerary status when fully realised has benefits (Wigens, 2004). However, the support for student nurses has to be balanced against the priority of care giving, and, therefore, support should be spread across the trained staff in the nursing team (Wigens, 2004). Learner support and confirmation of progress is not just the mentor's role but is seen as the role of the whole community of practice (Ohrling and Hallberg, 2001b; Phillips *et al.*, 2000a; Wigens, 2004). Individual learning becomes community learning through the process of disseminating and discussing individual knowledge within a team.

Evidence base

Read: Channell, W. (2002) Helping students to learn in the clinical environment. *Nursing Times*, **98**(39), 34–35.

Nurse education courses should look at current and future nursing practice and be assessed through work-based routes, such as portfolios of practice evidence. Classroom activities grounded in everyday situations recognise that knowledge is acquired in the situation and involves the social processes of thinking, perceiving and problem solving. Wenger (1998) suggests that the curriculum should be an itinerary of transformative experiences, maximising interactions – rather than just a list of subject matter. I agree with Wenger (1998) that using problem-based learning, reflecting on incidents and discussing the knowledge underpinning practice is more likely to be a transformative experience having longer-term significance than extensive coverage of broad, abstract and general curricula.

Academic and service partnerships

The current climate rewards universities and the NHS working together. Collaboration requires a closer partnership between lecturers, the HEI and the employers and services involved. However, having different 'communities of nurse academics' and 'communities of practitioners' means that these have distinct cultures (Mulhall, 2002). Practitioners consider that much of the research generated by academics asks irrelevant questions, lacks generalisation and has unrealistic resource implications (Mulhall, 2002), but academic–service partnerships that support the development of evidence-based practice are viewed as a fruitful area for collaboration. A research and evidence-based practice ethos needs to be championed at varying levels within organisations with forums for dissemination, such as specialist nurse link groups.

Evidence base

Take a look at Perry-Woodford, Z. and Whayman, K. (2005) Education in practice: a colorectal link-nurse programme. *British Journal of Nursing*, **14**(16), 862–866.

This article suggests that link nurses who attend an education programme and are given time to undertake this role have an increased awareness of the overall patient pathway and the role of the multidisciplinary team.

The implementation of research is strongly affected by clinical teams, requires 'old-timer' support, and needs to be applicable to the resource-constrained setting (Wigens, 2004). Nursing communities of practice find their own ways of connecting evidence-based knowledge to their everyday knowledge to achieve change. Nurses often read research evidence when they have access to it through CPD activities, as Thompson *et al.* (2001) found. Nurses also used oral story telling about poor practice in the past as a way of showing allegiance to evidence-based practice (Burke and Smith, 2000). Education courses or conferences may be the catalyst for a care change as they provide access to evidence from outside the nursing team. Senior nurses talk of 'pushing' to put evidence-based changes in place, a process which involves a transformation of the evidence into a context-sensitive form (Greenhalgh and Worrall, 1997). Facilitators of change need to know the context to justify their actions to others. Frameworks for evidence-based practice require sufficient flexibility for community interpretation within practice settings and are best developed within teams, either interprofessional or nursing specific as appropriate. Crucial to a 'learning culture' is the range of opportunities for discussion and debate about nursing practice.

Trust-wide frameworks can help embed evidence-based practice changes. A clinical guideline, for instance, can help a clinical team but the technical knowledge contained within a guideline still requires interpretation and has to be flexible enough 'in action' to be applicable to different clinical settings. There is less scepticism concerning guidelines and the possibility of these reducing professional practice (Stevens and Ledbetter, 2000) than might be expected, so long as guidelines are sufficiently flexible to fit into their 'real-world' setting (Eraut, 2000b). Opportunities for staff to see an evidence-based practice change working in another clinical area, or being used by a practitioner in their own clinical area, strengthen the chance of this change being adopted throughout a clinical setting. Using ideas and ways of working from other contexts can have a powerful impact on transforming practice.

As well as the academic–service partnerships created by evidence-based practice, the need for effective support of learners is also displayed when both the HEI and the placement provider are evaluated and quality assured in partnership in relation to health care educational programmes. The Department of Health established a multiprofessional quality assurance function for health care educational programmes within England in 2001. Following this, in 2003, a paper was published called *Streamlining Quality Assurance in Health Care Education. Purpose and Action* (DoH, 2003), which set out a rationale for the shape of a Partnership Quality Assurance Framework (PQAF). The 'partners' included health professional councils, the Department of Health, Strategic Health authorities and their associated NHS Trusts, and HEIs. The PQAF comprises five elements and is being developed for the Department of Health by Skills for Health. The elements are:

1   benchmarking and quality standards
2   programme approval
3   ongoing quality monitoring and enhancement (OQME)
4   major review
5   shared evidence base on which conclusions and judgements are based.

Self-and peer evaluation is undertaken, supported by evidence, to identify strengths and issues in relation to practice and campus learning, and action plans are proposed to improve the quality of education. The Quality Assurance Agency Major Review, which was completed in 2006, has provided a base line of peer review with the aims of:

- sharing good practice and innovation nationally
- assisting statutory bodies to maintain their obligations to protect the public
- providing evidence on the quality of higher education in health care provision, and
- ensuring that education is of a high quality for future employees.

Practice placements and campus-based learning are both quality assured as they are seen as integral to the whole health professional educational programme. The way that educational programmes are now quality assured acknowledges service providers' explicit role as practice educators. Quality assurance work to agree national standards is important to the wider policy initiative that has introduced a standard national framework contract for health care education. This has meant that the Department of Health gives the same benchmark price for each student of nursing wherever they undertake their training. It was also proposed that interdisciplinary funding of education should occur, ending the rigid demarcation of funding into different professional groups and allowing placement funding for all disciplines (DoH, 2002). This would be a major step forward but has not yet occurred.

The learning organisation

The Audit Commission (2001) suggests that it is necessary to engender a culture that values and expects training, learning and development. Over £3bn pounds are spent yearly on learning and professional development of health care staff in the NHS (DoH, 2002) so there needs to be sound justification for investing in continuing professional development (CPD). The quality of education is now being judged on its impact on practitioners' ability to deliver health services as part of a flexible competent workforce (DoH 1997). The importance of getting health professional education 'right' is an area of continuing debate. Levett-Jones (2005) suggests that CPD not only enhances knowledge and skills but there is also a positive correlation between professional development and staff satisfaction, staff retention and quality patient care. Nurses' ability to gain access to lifelong learning activities is aligned to retention in the clinical setting and, therefore, improved staffing levels. Mackereth (1989) found that staff felt valued if they had access to CPD and that this affected their morale, motivation and wish to stay within practice.

Over to you

- Locate and read a study-leave policy.
- Speak to three qualified health professional staff and ask them what training, education and continuous professional activities they have been involved with during the past year. Were there any differences in their ability to access CPD activities? If so, what were the reasons and how do you think this situation could be improved?

Study-leave policies need to be developed in consultation with staff, managers and professional bodies, and it is necessary to meet legal and statutory requirements. Managers should be made aware of the cost and significance of mistakes, in terms of education, training and development decisions, and how these mistakes can affect long- and short-term organisational priorities. An organisation's policy should aim to gain maximum benefit from education, and the policy should, therefore, identify priorities, encourage equity of training opportunities and give guidance to managers who are agreeing personal development plans. This can mean, however, that staff only have access to education that is regarded as organisationally high-priority; so one method used by some organisations for linking personal and organisational educational planning has been to offer annual credits for funding flexibility.

Increasing access to education and development is important, and guidelines for determining individual, directorate and Trust access to study leave should be transparent. Opportunities for education and training vary among different NHS Trusts (Audit Commission, 2001). Finding the time to undertake CPD activities can often be the biggest issue affecting access by health care professionals (Simons and Parry-Crooke, 2001). In one case site, there was variability in access to CPD activities between differing specialities within the same organisation (Wigens, 2004); this appeared to be linked to staffing levels and to the value placed on CPD by nurse leaders.

Training involves the systematic development of the knowledge, skills and attitudes required by an individual to perform a task or job adequately. An education strategy includes the processes for education and training within the workplace, which are regularly undertaken by an employing organisation, and should identify the way that education and training will be implemented, evaluated and audited over time. The strategy should link education and training activities to the priorities identified through business planning within the organisation (see Figure 10.1).

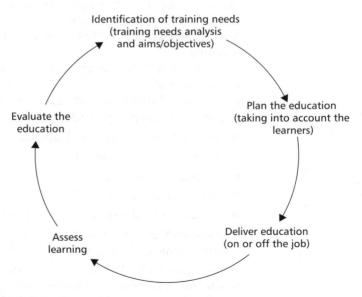

Figure 10.1 Education cycle

Range of factors driving an education strategy

The identification and analysis of training needs:

- Finance available – (scarce resources can be targeted, e.g. replacement finance for staff)
- New developments in the service
- The costs of study programmes (travel)
- Identification of available education (off the job) or the need for the creation of new education programmes based on learning objectives
- Format for the education, e.g. on the job – demonstration, coaching, rotation (planned experience), assignments or projects
- Improvements in staff knowledge and skills that are required
- The identification of key people who will be able to attend (can the education be interprofessional?)
- What benefits will be gained from the experience/education?
- How will staff pass on their knowledge and skills?
- Realistic timescales for completion

The NHS plan (DoH, 2000c) requires the modernisation of health care roles. This requires an organisation to have a broad span of activities in place to aid recruitment and retention, including mentorship, preceptorship and clinical supervision training, return to practice, international recruitment, NVQ training, flexible retirement, incentives and improved work practices. Healthy working conditions and an organisational culture where employees feel valued and have a common sense of loyalty can enhance retention of staff. By supporting a range of lifelong learning, an organisation can signal the value attached to learning.

A Training Needs Analysis (TNA) informs decision-making and is part of an education strategy. A TNA gives a baseline set of data to identify priorities and provides feedback on the effectiveness of previous decisions. Through the TNA:

- Learning objectives are established.
- Knowledge is mapped.
- Gaps are identified.
- Appropriate action is taken.
- Organisational issues are considered e.g. clinical developments.
- Data may be collected through questionnaires, observation, interviews and staff records.

Training needs analysis can be undertaken for an organisation as a whole, for departments or teams, or for individuals (sometimes the latter is called learning needs assessment [LNA]). Learning needs assessment is a part of TNA that assesses and understands an individual's needs through personal development planning (discussed within Chapter 5). Skilled contracting practices by Trusts, using best available data, assist organisations and their local education providers in ensuring that appropriate spending on education is targeted towards local priorities and staff needs.

The three basic methods for analysing education needs are:

- surveys and questionnaires to staff
- job analysis linked to the requirements for the job (e.g. KSF profile)
- personal development reviews.

The processes of TNA and LNA can be time consuming, and it can prove difficult to target specific areas, so the responsibility for delivering the education strategy is not just the employer's, but also the individual employee's. It is important that education is evaluated not only by seeing whether the objectives for the individual and the service area have been met but also whether the overall purpose has been achieved.

Kirkpatrick (1975) suggests that there are four levels of evaluation that can be undertaken with regard to education:

1 **reaction** – how the participants felt about the education; can be obtained through discussion, an evaluation sheet or questionnaire

2 **learning** – determining what skills and knowledge have been learnt through assessment

3 **behaviour** – observing the application of learning within the workplace

4 **results** – determining the effect on the organisation or the department of the education.

Reflective activity

Consider some education that you have received; this can be on or off the job. What was your immediate reaction to the education? What skills or knowledge did you gain as a result of this education that could be used in your practice? What level of evaluation was undertaken with regard to this education?

NHS Trusts should be lifelong learning organisations, making use of every opportunity to develop their staff, strengthening the image of the Trust as a 'good' employer. For example, there could be a structured plan for developing leadership skills throughout the organisation. The overall education, training and development strategy should reflect changes in work practices, team and individual needs, and local as well as national issues.

Educational roles

There are a number of educational roles that support learning within a health care organisation. In previous chapters, you will have looked at the mentor, preceptor, practice teacher and clinical supervisor roles. In this section, we examine other educational roles.

> ### Over to you
>
> Find out what educational posts are within your locality – some examples are listed here. Try to find out how to contact any of the following:
>
> - education and training leads (may be within a human resources, education or nursing department)
> - link lecturers
> - practice educators
> - trainers e.g. resuscitation, moving and handling
> - clinical practice facilitators
> - professional development nurses
> - work-based learning/NVQ co-ordinators.
>
> Ask at least two of these what they consider to be their main aims within their educational role.

Situated learning in practice can be fostered by educational roles; within this section these roles are broadly discussed under the title 'practice educator'. There are two models for practice educator implementation:

- the practice educator is based within the nursing/clinical team
- the practice educator visits a range of clinical areas.

If educational roles are sited within communities of practice, rather than educational facilitation being a visiting, auxiliary function, practice educators are more likely to play an integral part in the developing of personal development plans for staff members and formalised support structures. This can, however, be a costly model for practice education within an organisation, and visiting educational roles are, therefore, often used to enhance learning.

It is essential that practitioners are self-directed, but they must also appreciate the role of others as catalysts for their learning. Practice educators can act as critical companions helping practitioners to develop expertise, as they act as a resource and provide high levels of challenge and support (Manley *et al.*, 2005). External influences on the nursing teams are limited, so the role of these 'brokers' within communities of practice is important (Wenger, 1998). Brokers have multi-membership of communities of practice, and they help the transfer of practice from one community to another. They help create connections, but there is a fine balance between being seen as full members of one community and being rejected as an intruder in another. External facilitation by practice educators can allow staff to review the importance of the shared values that underpin current practice, without dictating a particular change in practice.

Human sources (clinically trusted and credible individuals) are overwhelmingly perceived as the most useful in reducing the uncertainties of nursing decisions (Thompson *et al.*, 2001). Clinical credibility is a necessary condition for perceiving a source of evidence, such as a practice educator, as useful. However, even though guidance is derived from others, one cannot assume that this has no basis in research knowledge.

A practice educator was asked about their role. Their responses have been summarised below.

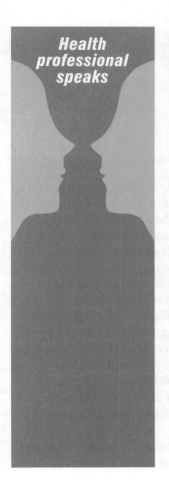

Health professional speaks

Practice educator

The advert for the Practice Development Nurse role was attractive to me because other institutions often want the person to be a full-time manager, full-time practitioner, as well as taking on this role. Senior staff try to take on this role, although they do not have the title, and the PDN role formalises this responsibility.

I saw my key objective was to 'Risk manage education within the department'– as there is a need to 'fit in' the education developments and identified education needs, requiring a commitment to prioritise covering staff time to access courses.

I make sure that I am visible on the 'shop floor'. If someone is off sick the staff are encouraged to try and seek a replacement, rather than to assume that the PDN will fill in, but if there is a crisis I will work with a member of staff in a mentoring role. When working with staff there is questioning and coaching regarding practice as the care is delivered.

When there are vacancies, especially at a senior level within a department/ward, there can be a constant battle between the PDN role and function and service needs. This can cause a 'guilty conscience' that you cannot stop – it is always there, although the PDN needs to maintain clinical credibility. I meet up with two other PDNs to receive group clinical supervision, and balancing the need to facilitate learning and cover care delivery are constantly coming up as an issue.

The team days I arrange are not viewed as 'optional' and good rostering is the key. To encourage people to attend, there need to be visible benefits (e.g. development of Patient Group Directives). Study days are easier to plan for, as you cannot take people out for an hour at a time as this affects the service. The PDN needs to ensure that they do not de-skill those interested in the facilitation of learning. For instance, one of the staff continues to co-ordinate the mentorship of student nurses, whilst the PDN in this case focuses on registered staff and support staff.

The practice educator talking in the last excerpt had a dedicated educational role. Field (2004) has suggested that practice educators may be clinically and academically competent, but that their lack of constant clinical engagement can mean that they have less clinical expertise when compared with mentors and clinical supervisors. A learning organisation is likely to invest in dedicated educational roles as well as in those who integrate support of practice-based learning with a defined clinical workload.

Nurse teachers, too, have a role in supporting learning in practice. The NMC states that 20% of the normal teaching hours of nurse teachers should be taken up with supporting learning in practice (NMC, 2006). This can be done in many ways.

Nurse teacher activities to support learning through practice

- Acting as a link lecturer
- Supporting mentor and practice teacher development
- Active clinical role
- Professional and practice development
- Contributing to practice research
- Involvement in action learning sets
- Supporting clinical leadership development

Finding an appropriate role for the nurse teacher within practice, as well as higher education, has created some difficulties. The role of the nurse teacher has been perceived as becoming more 'academic' and less committed to nursing practice (Crotty, 1993), and some students have become dissatisfied with the type and frequency of their interactions with the nurse teachers. There is a need for clarification of the current confusion regarding the clinical role of nurse lecturers and for nurse lecturers to have an active presence in practice settings, maintaining their clinical knowledge and credibility (Ioannides, 1999). Educational activities can only be directly related to practice if nurse lecturers have a strong working relationship with clinical practice. If nurse educators are to function as facilitators of learning, they need to identify their role within practice or they will be unable to show authenticity in their subject matter (Wigens, 2004). Nurse teachers can facilitate practice-based learning, and practice educator roles can also cross over into higher education with mutual benefit.

The NMC teacher standard, which applies to practice educators and nurse teachers who support learning in practice and academic environments, requires them to have at least three years' post-registration experience on the same part of the professional register as the learners they support. They should hold a first degree and an approved teacher preparation post-graduate qualification (this is usually a year-long course which involves 360 hours assessed teaching) (NMC, 2006).

Evidence base

The NMC postgraduate teacher qualification is also recognised by the Higher Education National Academy (HENA) which specifies that evidence of teaching activities, core/specialist knowledge and professional values are necessary to meet the national standard (HENA, 2006).

Take a look at the following website: www.heacademy.ac.uk

Practice educators require support, just like students and junior colleagues, but have a tendency to focus on meeting the needs of students and their mentors, neglecting their own professional support requirements. Nurses in senior roles who are helping to support learning through practice may be quite isolated and may find that educational and professional support mechanisms are lacking. A new nurse teacher often has an identified mentor who is an experienced educator. However, as time progresses there is often no formalised support role identified and it is tacitly expected that teachers will develop their own educational support network, outside the usual academic line management. Stress levels can be high within education, with the general pressures of academic life being compounded by schemes to assess the quality of teaching and research (Ioannides, 1999). A nurse lecturer can benefit from an identified clinical colleague who acts as a clinical support to the lecturer.

Peer clinical supervision may be in place for practice educators; however, this can be reduced by the everyday fluctuations in supervisory and teaching workloads. Cushen and Wigens (2000) advocate the setting up of transformational partnerships between lecturers, practice educators and senior clinical nurses, whereby nurses working in different organisations or specialities can provide mutual clinical support. This partnership can assist professional and personal development as well as giving time out to reflect on practice. A transformational partnership should be an equal relationship, where peers work together in a collegiate fashion, empowering partners to work to their full potential, by challenging current working and encouraging a sense of direction. There has to be respect and understanding of each other's unique perspective on learning through practice.

Fostering communities of practice

I have suggested in preceding chapters that learning is context sensitive. The progression of learning within nursing is likely to reflect national changes in health care practice. This will involve movement from a traditional, hierarchical situation, in which theory is front-loaded, and patient involvement is limited and routinised, to one where nursing is collegiate, understanding of theories is developed within practice and sufficient effort is made to engage with patients over care decisions. There is considerable support for NHS Trusts to develop as learning organisations (DoH, 1997), but there has been less explicit acceptance or support for the development of communities of practice and situated learning. Matthews and Candy (1999) estimate that perhaps 90% of organisational learning occurs incidentally or adventitiously, through exposure to the opinions and practices of others also working in the same context.

Wenger and colleagues' (2002) exploration of the relationships of communities of practice to official organisations identified five main relationships (previously discussed in Chapter 4). Nursing teams mainly reach level 3 ('legitimised' within the organisation). Levels 4 or 5 ('strategic' and 'transformative') might be achieved by fostering nursing and interprofessional teams as central to learning within NHS organisations. However, understandably, the educational and learning function of nursing teams is often seen as secondary to care delivery. It would be helpful, therefore, for these two crucial functions to be viewed as inextricably related. Wenger *et al.* (2002) emphasise the relationship between resources and the creating of a learning environment, as without adequate resources the learning environment can be patchy. Their seven goals for a learning organisation are:

- designing for evolution
- having an open dialogue with varying levels of participation
- developing public and private community spaces
- focusing on value
- combining familiarity
- excitement
- a rhythm for learning (Wenger *et al.*, 2002, p. 51).

As discussed in Chapter 9, nursing communities play a powerful part in coping with resource and other constraints. The constant care delivery functions of nursing teams and the resource constraints under which they operate mean that they lack many of the formal structures to facilitate reflective learning, focusing instead on crisis management. If time and resources for learning are to be found, it is necessary to make explicit the factors that will help this to be achieved. Working patterns are presently determined by patient care workload, but appreciating that staff need time to engage with others and factoring this into staffing rotas is an example of a practical approach to cultivating a learning environment. Managers could benefit from awareness of the status of team development so that they do not over-manage teams or inadvertently penalise the work involved in building the community (Wenger *et al.*, 2002).

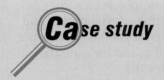

Case study

Strengthening teamworking

The breast care clinical team had been dissatisfied with the way that their multidisciplinary working was going. There was a perception that not all members of the team were clear about the recent changes in practice. It was agreed that as many as could be freed from practice commitments would get together for a 'team building and agreeing the vision' workshop day. The breast care nurse specialist, Alexandra, had spent a considerable amount of her own time planning this and had worked hard, with colleagues, to plan for a good attendance and a structure so that future working could be based on the action plan that came out of the day. The day before the workshop Alexandra's service manager asked Alexandra to cancel the event, as there were difficulties in staffing some of the wards in their directorate and all education and development was to be cancelled.

Do you feel that the service manager's decision was appropriate? How do you think Alexandra should handle this request?

When 'newcomers' arrive and 'old-timers' leave, there is an impact on the learning environment and on teamwork. Experienced nurses can offer up past patient care experiences as 'packages of situated knowledge', making their practice meaningful to others (Wigens, 2004). Nurses may perceive themselves as lacking control over work practices and workload, and active involvement in strategy and policy development from 'grass roots' staff should be sought. Like the psychotherapists studied by Dreier (1996), some nurses have an 'exaggerated sense' of the extent to which external changes are imposed upon them (Wigens, 2004), and this can lead to reliance on restricted and individualised coping strategies. Those involved in supporting learning through practice should challenge this perception.

Burgoyne (1994) makes explicit reference to policy making, strategy, evaluation, and learner rewards as influential factors in organisational learning. Both Burgoyne (1994) and Wenger *et al.* (2002) identify 'change' or 'excitement' as facets of a learning environment. The rapid pace of change in health care may act as a constant source of pressure that potentially overloads practitioners, or as an opportunity for professional development. Nurses need to be involved as stakeholders in owning the changes that affect their practice so that new, expanded and re-engineered roles can be integrated into the team through the mutual re-evaluation of 'nursing work' (Wigens, 2004). A clinical career ladder is crucial to retaining nurses in practice and to meeting service objectives, and a co-ordinated approach to instigating new posts, such as nurse consultant, clinical lead nurses, and specialist nurse and nurse practitioner roles, is necessary.

There is sometimes a rather ad hoc approach to decisions about access to CPD (Wigens, 2004), and a learning organisation must make appraisal and personal development planning priorities, if CPD for staff is to be co-ordinated. Keeping a professional portfolio to meet individual, as well as professional body, requirements can be emphasised and supported through in-house education about portfolio development and reflective writing. Decisions to undertake formal educational courses are based on a mixture of practice, personal work and academic aspirations, and a supportive learning environment appreciates this.

Leadership sets the overall direction for education and learning. Nolan and colleagues (1995) found that managers wanted to see a greater impact from CPD activities that their staff had attended but may have failed to provide an environment in which change or 'social capital' can flourish. At present, mentors and preceptors may carry unrealistic workloads, leaving little time for learner support (Edmond, 2001). The clinical teaching commitment for practitioners is usually unrecognised and undervalued, and the requisite time and resources are seldom allocated (Eraut *et al.*, 1998). Rolfe (1993) argues that less time should be spent on applying theories to practice and more time should be allocated to reflection on individual clinical situations and to reflective diaries, portfolios and critical incident work. Time needs to be available for personal reflection and self-assessment within professional practice. Opportunities to debrief and reflect on practice helped learners to learn through their practice, and make and articulate the links between theory and practice.

✍ *Over to you*

Find out about the leadership and management education and CPD activities related to leadership development available in your organisation.

According to a number of theorists (Harvey *et al.*, 2002; Wenger *et al.*, 2002) a key factor in setting up and promoting a successful community of practice is the vitality of the leadership. Time and funding to undertake the leadership and co-ordinating function for a community are important, and senior nurses require 'ring-fenced' time for this crucial role (Wigens, 2004). Situated leadership in nursing comes from a credible clinical base and a visible presence. Situated leadership can be diverse and there is no definitive style of leadership. Flexible leaders engage with, filter and transform different forms of evidence, so that within a community of practice a sense of shared understanding and ownership of what the leader and overall organisation are trying to accomplish can be achieved. However, healthy communities do not depend entirely on one person for leadership. Developing others and having the 'right' people in place is also part of the facilitation of learning. A 'facilitating culture' is one in which clinical leaders are committed to their own, and others', lifelong learning (Wigens, 2004).

Situated leadership involves the balancing of communal memory with change, as well as being able to share visions and values in a collective and supportive way (Stordeur *et al.*, 2001). Leaders have a 'scaffolding effect' (Rogoff, 1990), offering a mature arena for learners. An interaction between team members, such as outlining what care has been given or a change in care for a patient, can include a hidden request for teaching, and where relationships are mature this can be the starting point for further learning (Wigens, 2004). The subtlety of these requests is perhaps linked to a reluctance to appear inexperienced in front of patients and student nurses (Wigens, 2004). The response from experienced staff to these 'disguised' requests can be variable but usually takes the form of additional information and of senior staff making themselves available to those undertaking a new practice. Nurses should be open about their need for further practice-based learning and not see this as something that will weaken their professionalism in the eyes of others.

The nursing team acts as a social network or 'framework' for professional practice and learning, and nursing practice is enabled by the development of community of practice processes that include:

- fostering a 'facilitative culture'
- developing situated leadership
- encouraging lifelong learning and continuous professional development
- utilising prioritisation frameworks
- implementing situated changes
- combining care activities
- sustaining communal memory
- reducing dissonance and conflict
- making personal learning explicit.

Professional practice is learnt through shared work and the sharing of narratives, and through reflecting, interpreting and negotiating as nurses represent their social world. Theories-in-use, such as the valuing of visibility within clinical areas and maintaining clinical credibility at a senior level, and the mental frameworks used for prioritising patient care are examples of theorising practice identified within one study (Wigens, 2004).

A thorough grasp of the clinical setting is a requirement for effective clinical decision-making for all those involved in a community of practice, and its mastery requires a composite of skills. In fact, the speed of care delivery and decision-making demonstrated by experienced staff can sometimes be perceived by others as showing an uncaring or blasé approach to patient care (Wigens, 2004). In such circumstances, experienced nurses who are able to talk openly about their day-to-day decision-making, sharing their insights and experiences, can find meaning in these interactions. When nurses are encouraged to discuss their judgements in a daily context in an open and constructive manner, not just in response to adverse events, they can start to determine how they form skilled and expert judgements.

Decisions are often made within nursing through the sharing of information and in discussion with others; this is not a weakness in professional clinical decision-making, but a sign of a 'community of practice' in action. Decisions are rarely clear cut and made with a full knowledge base; therefore, the support of others, evinced through questioning and searching quickly for information, helps to manage uncertainty. When shift timings and staffing levels are being considered, attempts to instigate or maintain times for learning and debate on working practices, such as team meetings and action learning sets, should be supported.

Working at a fast pace can be a way of accommodating time for difficult patient situations that might occur but has an impact on the quality of the nurse–patient relationship. Dreier (1996, p. 115) suggests that psychotherapists need to think beyond the immediate situation and locate their interaction within the 'structure of the client's lifeworld'; many nurses also mention this (Wigens, 2004). An open dialogue with patients aimed at improving patient care requires experienced nurses to get feedback from patients. Experienced nurses who use these sorts of approaches to feedback as well as survey data, such as the national patient survey, can act as role models for others.

Reflective activity

Think about one clinical area. How much engagement was there between the health care practitioners and the patients/clients? What part did the team leaders play in this?

Learning must be personally meaningful, as motivation, activity and learning are related to positive self-esteem and identity, and the individual nurse is shaped by their relationship to their community of practice. Membership of a nursing community is inextricably linked with individual motivations to nurse and engagement through development of a 'professional identity'. Opportunities for reflection and analysis of practice and development of professional identity can be supported by formal learning structures such as mentorship, preceptorship, clinical supervision and interprofessional networking time. Dialogue, as a means of sharing information, ideas and feelings, is vital for collective learning (Phillips, 1994). If learning is viewed as more than an individual process, then what enables the social process of learning is 'space' – time for reflection, questions, review, permission to be open and say the 'unsayable', and support (Phillips, 1994, p. 100). The formal structures for reflecting on practice and professional issues can combine with informal support networks to promote a 'facilitating culture'. For transformation to take place, what is required is just enough structure to provide safe conditions and space in which people can change.

If the 'virtual space' away from direct patient care is to be provided for nurses to take up learning support activities, network, and shadow others, NHS organisations have to value these learning activities. Physical space is also required for learning activities such as clinical supervision meetings, and this can be a practical problem for nursing teams. Where possible, learning areas need to be identified; access to break areas near to the working spaces of nurses, but private from patients, can help in the development of team spirit. Social interactions (time to laugh, moan and have fun) are a vital part of a well-functioning community of practice.

In advocating that clinical teams are fostered as communities of practice, I have predominantly aligned myself with the view of professional working as 'professional artistry' rather than 'technical rationalism' (Fish and Coles, 1998). Technical rationality is based on instrumental problem-solving made rigorous by the application of specialised, firmly bounded, scientific and standardised professional knowledge (Schön, 1983). Currently, there is a movement towards technical rationalism within the NHS that could be seen as a 'backlash' against the previous professional artistry approach to health care practice. Competence frameworks (popular within nursing and health care at present) can drive the range of experiences and skills progression. Those committed to the technical rationalist viewpoint might suggest that my ideas for fostering communities of practice and situated, holistic learning in nursing are insufficiently specific. However, new competences and enhanced skill developments have their meaning negotiated within the community of practice and 'old-timers' have to work to keep up with new practices. Part of this process involves the partnership that occurs when experienced nurses are supervising 'new comers' (e.g. students, newly qualified staff, international recruits, and new staff to a speciality) and this important facilitation role requires recognition organisationally.

From a 'professional artistry' perspective, practice involves a blending of practitioner qualities, skills, metacognitive awareness and creative imagination processes that allows 'self' to be used in professional work (RCN, 2002b). Reflective practice is about professional artistry and offers a model for dealing with complexity, uniqueness and the realities of professional practice (Schön, 1983) and is inclusive of evidence-based practice. The constant dialogue between thought and action in professional artistry involves social relationships that can be fostered within nursing teams. Critiques might indicate that, although professional artistry has been advocated for some considerable time, little change has actually occurred. This is perhaps not surprising, as I have identified many infrastructural facets to cultivating the context within which communities of practice will thrive. These include informal and formal support for learning at an individual level (e.g. clinical supervision), at nursing team level (e.g. evidence-based change in practice project), and at an organisational level (e.g. stakeholder involvement in educational policy and strategy development). The challenge is to manage the dance between formal and informal learning (Wenger *et al.*, 2002).

Throughout this book there has been a central tension between the view that all learning is socially based (discussed in Chapters 3, 4 and 9) and the importance placed on individualistic aspects of personal learning (explored particularly in Chapters 2, 5, 6, and 7). The same clinical setting can provoke very different learning, and different nursing teams vary in their clinical learning environments. The centre of nurses' learning seems to be located in their professional and personal identities, as well as in their relationships and the situation. Within this book, I have tried to handle the problem of integrating individual perspectives of learning, such as reflection, into situated learning theories. In a similar way to Billett (2001), I see nurses in a dialogic association with their workplace relationships, with mutual interactions changing both; however, I do not see a nurse and a community of practice as independent. Individual nurses are part of a nursing team but are also separate from the nursing team. Nursing identities are built and grounded in practice activities. I have, therefore, addressed a range of elements that could optimise learning through practice. These include making explicit the different forms of knowledge used in practice, allocating time to teach, support and discuss practice with colleagues, teamworking, effective leadership and communication, and the management of change.

RRRRR**Rapid recap**

Check your progress in learning from this book and from this last chapter by working through each of the following questions.

1   Give four teaching methods that could help to integrate theory and practice.
2   Why are academic and service partnerships being encouraged?
3   What reasons could a learning organisation give for encouraging the continuous professional development of its employees?
4   What is a training needs analysis?
5   What activities may a nurse teacher undertake within a clinical setting?
6   List at least four community-of-practice processes that can occur in nursing teams.

If you have difficulty with one of these questions, read through the section again to refresh your understanding.

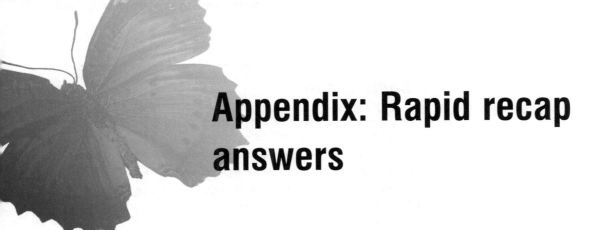

Appendix: Rapid recap answers

Chapter 1

1 What is situated learning?

Situated learning takes place in the setting where the learning will be applied, and assumes that social processes will affect this learning.

2 What is a community of practice?

A community of practice is where learning is seen as an act of membership and participation in a social group that integrates knowledge and situated learning into its life and working.

3 Define the term 'tacit knowledge'.

Tacit knowledge is rooted in context, people, places, ideas and experiences. A person carries tacit knowledge around in their mind from their experience; they may not consciously be aware of it, but it helps them to undertake their daily tasks.

4 Give some examples of evidence that could be used within a professional portfolio.

The range of evidence that can be offered to indicate learning through practice includes portfolios and profiles, reflective accounts, critical incident analyses, career biographies, learning diaries and competencies and skills documentation.

Chapter 2

1 What are the key differences between outcome-based and process-based learning?

The key differences between outcome- and process-based learning are that outcome-based learning is based on knowledge taken in and absorbed by the learner and retained for future use. It uses a building block approach, where knowledge is accumulated. Process-based learning involves a flexible network of ideas, knowledge and feelings, where learning involves a process of assembling, ordering or modifying understanding (termed assimilation by Piaget, 1971). Learning as a process is seen as grounded in experience, requiring a resolution of conflicts between alternative ways of looking at and adapting to the world. It involves transactions between the learner and the environment and leads to the creation of knowledge.

2 List the key principles underpinning:

(a) behaviourist theories of learning

(b) cognitive theories of learning

(c) humanistic theories of learning.

The key principles underpinning the following types of learning are:

Behaviourist – from a behaviourist stance, learning is the result of the application of consequences i.e. learners begin to connect certain responses with certain stimuli. There are two components to learning – Stimulus>Response. Different behavioural theories elaborate on this basic paradigm. Within the classical conditioning model, learning starts with an unconditioned response to an unconditioned (positive or negative) stimulus, a reflex. Other models focus on the consequences of the action, whether pleasant or otherwise. This adds another component to learning – Stimulus>Response>Outcome. An environmental event (for example a patient having a cardiac arrest) may act as a stimulus, and the outcome of the individual's response to the stimulus can be either negative or positive. Reinforcement will lead to a change in behaviour, either to increase or decrease the likelihood of the behaviour recurring.

Cognitive learning is seen as coming from experience, reasoning and remembering information that allows the person to adapt to the environment. Learning involves the act of knowing, discovering and making meaning through intellectual processing and mental structuring. Understanding learning requires the study of information processing, as learning requires varying levels of elaboration moving from perception to the making of meaning. Remembering can be enhanced when, through experience, a person adds more connections to a single concept.

Humanistic learning is focused on personal growth, the development of self-direction and interpersonal relationships. Behaviours are viewed as intentional and based on values, so to understand learning from this stance we need to study a person holistically as they grow and develop throughout their life. Feedback about learning is internal to the 'self' and based on individual motivations, goal setting and areas of interest.

3 Explain the concepts 'lifelong learning' and 'continuous professional development'.

Explanations of lifelong learning and continuing professional development are as follows:

Lifelong learning has been defined as a process of accomplishing personal, social and professional development throughout the lifespan of the individual in order to enhance the quality of life of individuals and groups. It makes an assumption that learning takes place in all spheres of life, not just within educational institutes or in educational programmes.

Continuous professional development is a range of learning activities through which professionals maintain and develop knowledge and expertise throughout their career to ensure that they retain their capacity to practise safely, effectively and legally within their evolving scope of practice.

4 Why is it useful to be able to document learning through practice?

It is useful to be able to document learning through practice because this can demonstrate to others a level of knowledge, competence or working. A student who is being assessed in relation to their practice learning will need to document their learning through practice to show how their theoretical and practical learning have become integrated. A qualified member of staff will document learning through practice evidence to demonstrate CPD achievement and a level of practice required to undertake their clinical role.

Chapter 3

1 Define the term 'reality shock' and identify the possible stages of this.

'Reality shock' is the term used for conflict caused by, for example, the movement from the familiar higher education environment to the unfamiliar work setting, caused by a gap between what has been learnt and on-the-job experiences.

The possible stages of reality shock are:

- Honeymoon – the student is fascinated with the new work.
- Shock/Rejection – the student rejects the new environment, or the old environment, or self and may become socially isolated.
- Recovery – the student is able to see the funny side of this, and is becoming competent.
- Resolution – the student is able to display culturally appropriate reactions.

2 What should be the minimum number of formal meetings that a mentor/supervisor undertakes with a student, and what structure could be used for these meetings?

The minimum number of formal meetings that a mentor/supervisor undertakes with a student should be three.

A possible structure for these meetings would be as follows:

- Think about the introduction and purpose of the meeting.
- Take time to put the learner at ease.
- Explain how the meeting will be recorded.
- Ask generally about how it is going.
- Ask about their practice learning, work/study patterns and if they have any problems.
- Review their assessment work so far.
- Deal with any specific issues the learner wants to raise.
- Discuss the arrangements for follow-up/further meetings.

3 How should a student handle a period of sickness or absence from a placement area?

A student should handle a period of sickness or absence from a placement area by informing the clinical staff prior to the start of the shift and also the higher education institute.

4 What guidance does the QAAHE think should be made available to all students attending a placement area?

The QAAHE believes that placements need to be effectively prepared for student allocation and should provide equitable opportunity for each individual to achieve their respective placement outcomes. Institutions should ensure that students are provided with appropriate guidance and support in preparation for, during and after their placements, which includes:

- appropriate induction to the placement environment including health and safety information
- any occupational health, legal or ethical considerations or requirements (e.g. patient confidentiality)
- the means of recording the achievement of learning outcomes
- availability of additional skills preparation
- cultural orientation and work expectations
- institutional support services that students can access.

Chapter 4

1 What types of student–patient relationship may be developed within a clinical learning environment?

The types of student-patient relationship that may be developed within a clinical learning environment are mechanistic, authoritative and facilitative.

2 Define the 'hidden curriculum' within health care professional education.

The 'hidden curriculum' within health care professional education means the unacknowledged, covert socialising processes of education that lead to the learning of cultural norms, values and beliefs.

3 What, in the view of Weidman *et al.* (2001), are the four components of professional socialisation?

In Weidman, Twale and Stein's (2001) view, the four components of professional socialisation are:

- prospective students (background, predisposition)

- professional communities (practitioners, associations)
- personal communities (family, friends and employers)
- novice professional practitioners.

4 Explain in your own words the following concepts:
  (a) legitimate peripheral participation
  (b) communal memory
  (c) professional artistry.

Any explanations of the following concepts which are broadly similar to the examples below would be appropriate:

(a) legitimate peripheral participation – this is where a student works within a community of practice, learning about the working of the clinical setting without full team membership

(b) communal memory – this is the memory of events held by 'old timers' within a community of practice, e.g. how things have changed so much as the matrons are not strict like they used to be

(c) professional artistry – this is the way an expert practitioner determines the delivery of their care, not just basing this on clinical guidelines or care routines.

5 Identify five factors that help the development of a community of practice clinical team.

Factors that help the development of a community of practice clinical team are:

- Individuals learn and gain confidence by contributing to communities of practice.
- Communities are able to refine their practice whilst ensuring continued membership.
- The team transfer knowledge and skills throughout the membership.
- The clinical team can help staff invent and maintain ways of coping with the shifting 'real world' situation.
- The clinical team is able to use the process of legitimate peripheral participation to bring new members into the group whilst achieving continuity.
- Knowledge acquired in the authentic context has better chance of being activated when needed in another situation.
- Communities of practice are forums for situated knowledge and can assist in resolving conflict.

6 List three possible problems with relying on community of practice processes for clinical learning.

Three possible problems with relying on community of practice processes for clinical learning are:

- Like other people, nurses and other health care practitioners do not seem to be able to impart the knowledge they have.

- There is often a level of conflict between staff which can affect learning.

- Nursing practice can remain unchallenged and can stagnate.

Chapter 5

1 Identify a minimum of four factors that are likely to affect an individual's learning.

Four factors that are likely to affect an individual's learning are: motivation, personal life situation, employer support in providing either funding or study leave, and the learner's individual personality and learning style.

2 What is a reason for finding out someone's learning style? Give the names of two models that could be used to do this.

A reason for finding out someone's learning style is to enable them to become more motivated to learn by knowing more about their own strengths and weaknesses.

Models that could be used to do this are: the Dunn and Dunn Model; The Myers-Briggs Type Indicator (MBTI); Kolb's Learning Style Inventory (LSI) and Honey and Mumford's Learning Styles.

3 What are the characteristics of information that can be used to help in the successful development of a learning objective?

In order to develop a successful learning objective, ensure that the information you have should be **S**MART, i.e:

S P E C I F I C

M E A S U R A B L E

A C H I E V A B L E

R E A L I S T I C

T I M E B O U N D.

4 What are the core dimensions of the NHS KSF and the role and responsibilities of an appraisee?

The core dimensions of the NHS KSF are communication; personal and people development; health, safety and security; service improvement; development; quality; equality and diversity.

The role and responsibilities of an appraisee are to: understand the KSF outline for their post; evaluate their achievements referring to the KSF outline; identify their strengths; gather and structure evidence that demonstrates their achievements; identify their learning and development needs; prioritise, identify and arrange training and development activities to meet their learning needs; identify their personal contribution towards their personal development plan.

5 Identify the five key components of a learning contract or a personal development plan.

The five key components of a learning contract or a personal development plan are:

- the knowledge, skills, attitudes, and values to be acquired by the learner (learning objectives)

- how these objectives are to be accomplished by the learner (learning resources and strategies)

- the target date(s) for completion

- what evidence will be presented to demonstrate that the objectives have been completed (evidence of accomplishment)

- how this evidence will be judged or validated (criteria and means for validating evidence) (Knowles, 1986).

Chapter 6

1 What are the main differences between mentorship and preceptorship?

The main differences between mentorship and preceptorship are:

A mentor:

- facilitates learning, supervises and assesses students during their clinical placements (usually around a 10–12 weeks' placement)

- is required to have successfully completed a Preparation for Mentorship qualification, usually at Level 3 (Hons degree) in order to undertake this role.

A preceptor:

- supports the growth and development of a novice registered practitioner
- fulfils this role for a fixed and limited amount of time with the specific purpose of assisting the novice into their new role (often 4–6 months)
- helps with the socialising of new team members into a practice community, helping them to become full members of the team.

2   How should a mentor handle a situation where a student is performing poorly and is at risk of failing their practice assessment in the placement?

When a student is performing poorly and is at risk of failing their practice assessment in the placement, a mentor should be honest, providing constructive feedback. The mentor should also seek the support of the educational institute link person to ensure that they are aware of the poor performance and impending referral if the student does not improve in line with an agreed action plan.

3   What issues need to be decided in order to formalise a preceptorship programme?

In order to formalise a preceptorship programme, the following need to be agreed:

- the role of the preceptor, the relationship of the preceptor and preceptee within a preceptorship programme
- who requires preceptorship – for newly qualified staff, those returning from breaks in service and those returning after working for a significant time in a very different speciality
- the format for guidelines/documentation of the preceptorship period
- practical issues, training and support resources available, and how this differs from current arrangements

4   Define 'clinical supervision' and name two models/frameworks for clinical supervision.

Clinical supervision is a formal process with a skilled supervisor and supervisee. It should enable a professional to reflect on and assume responsibility for their practice, develop skills, knowledge and understanding of their practice whilst feeling supported. It is advocated for all clinical practitioners as it enhances consumer protection and safety of care in increasingly complex clinical situations.

Models/ frameworks for clinical supervision are:

Wagner's (1957) supervision triangle, Heron's (1989) six-category intervention analysis, Proctor's (1987) three-function interactive model , Stoltenberg and Delworth's (1987) integrative development model

5   Why are ground rules necessary within clinical supervision?

Ground rules are necessary within clinical supervision to ensure that practitioners and supervisors are aware of what is involved and can trust in the confidentiality of clinical supervision.

Chapter 7

1   How does experiential learning differ from classroom-based traditional teaching?

Experiential learning differs from classroom-based traditional teaching as it encourages deep, rather than surface, approaches to learning. It is rooted in 'doing' and purposeful reflection, which gives meaning to experience and enables the discovery of knowledge that may not be evident through everyday experience alone.

2   List three frameworks that can guide reflection.

Three frameworks that can guide reflection are: Gibbs' reflective cycle structured reflection model; Palmer, Burns and Bulman's reflective framework; Johns' (2000) model of structured reflection.

3   What are the stages of the adapted Gibbs' reflective cycle?

The six stages of Gibbs' reflective cycle are: description, action plan, feelings, evaluation, conclusion and analysis.

4   Define problem-based learning and action learning?

Problem-based learning reflects the way people learn in real life, as they tend simply to get on with solving the problems life puts before them with whatever resources are to hand.

Action learning is the application of the experiential learning cycle to work activities and is designed to improve practice by basing future decisions and actions on the learning that has occurred through discussing practice with others.

5 What stages are there in making an evidence-based change in practice?

The stages in making an evidence-based change in practice are:

- Identify an area of practice.
- Undertake a literature review.
- Discuss the available literature with colleagues.
- Agree 'best practice' with colleagues.
- Compare 'best practice' to current practice.
- Make a change in practice if necessary.
- Evaluate the new practice.

Chapter 8

1 What are the key differences between:

    (a) formative and summative assessment of practice

    (b) criterion-referenced and norm-referenced assessment of practice?

(a) The key differences between formative and summative assessment of practice are:

- Formative assessment takes place throughout the placement and is an informal assessment where the 'marks' do not count towards the final result. This type of assessment helps to identify strengths and weaknesses, and the level of student learning and progress. The assessor can use the formative assessment to identify a need for further explanation, additional practice experience, or whether learning can move on to other areas.

- Summative assessment usually takes place at the end of a placement and is a formal assessment where the 'mark' is used to determine the level of achievement. It can determine how much has been learnt by the student and the extent to which the learning outcomes have been met.

(b) The key difference between criterion- referenced and norm-referenced assessment of practice is that criterion-referenced assessment relies on the explicit criteria provided by the education institute in order to make an assessment, whereas norm referencing compares students who are at the same stage of training and looks at how each is progressing compared with others in the group.

2 What are the level identifiers within Steinaker and Bell's (1979) experiential taxonomy?

The level identifiers within Steinaker and Bell's (1979) experiential taxonomy are:

- Exposure – the student has observed the skill being performed by a competent practitioner.
- Participation – the student has assisted a competent practitioner in the performance of the skill.
- Identification – the student has performed the skill under the supervision of a registered practitioner.
- Internalisation – the student has sustained a skilled performance in a variety of settings under the supervision of a registered practitioner.
- Dissemination – the student has maintained professional competence and has enabled others to develop their knowledge and skills.

3 Identify at least six forms of evidence that could be included within a practice portfolio.

Forms of evidence that could be included within a practice portfolio are: observation of practical skills, student self assessment, discussion, learning contracts, guided study, written reflection, testimony of others, interviews, patient comments and feedback, peer evaluation, audit or data collection, case study, team project.

4 What are the five levels that Benner (1984) identified regarding the development of nursing expertise?

The five levels that Benner (1984) identified regarding the development of nursing expertise are:

Level 1: Novice – Beginners have had no experience of the situation. There may be rigid adherence to taught rules and plans, little situational perception, no discretionary judgement.

Level 2: Advanced Beginner – Demonstrates marginally acceptable performance, using guidelines for action, based on attributes or aspects; situational perceptions still limited; all attributes and aspects are treated separately and given equal importance.

Level 3: Competent – Has been in similar situations and begins to see his/her actions in terms of the 'bigger' picture. Coping with many forms of information, sees actions partly in terms of long-term goals, conscious planning, standardised and routinised procedures.

Level 4: Proficient – Perceives situations as a whole and demonstrates a 'smooth' clinical performance. Sees what is most important in a situation, perceives deviations from the normal, decision-making less laboured.

Level 5 Expert – No longer relying on principles, rules or guidelines to connect their actions to the appropriate situation. Intuitive grasp of situations based on tacit understanding, analytical approaches only used in novel situations or where problems occur, have a vision of what is possible.

5   What should be done about patient information, when placing evidence that links to patient care practice into an assessment-of-practice document?

When placing evidence that links to patient care practice into an assessment of practice document, patient information should be removed as patient confidentially should be maintained at all times.

Chapter 9

1   What strategies may nurses use to cope with high workloads, time pressures and information overload?

The strategies that nurses may use to cope with high workloads, time pressures and information overload are:

- speeding up (acceleration)
- selecting the input of information (filtering)
- prioritising
- using 'decision rules'
- omitting or avoiding
- locking on to one approach.

2   What three phases do Crawford and Kiger (1998) suggest students progress through whilst on clinical placement?

The three phases that Crawford and Kiger (1998) suggest that students progress through whilst on clinical placement are:

- adaptation (becoming part of the community)
- stabilisation (increased knowledge and skills)
- consolidation (requiring reduced supervision.

3   Outline the main aspects of the four models of practitioner-patient relationship.

The main aspects of the four models of practitioner–patient relationship are:

(a) Nurse centred – This model influenced nursing in the past, and emphasised dependence of the patient on the health carer. Care giving was determined by the nurse who was viewed as more 'knowledgeable' than the patient. Care was delivered, it was perceived, in the patient's best interest.

(b) Technical relationship – Nursing is seen as a clinical science, where skilled, objective care is delivered without imposing any of the carer's values or wishes. In this model, the nurse's responsibility predominantly revolves around his or her technical competence. The patient may have the ultimate responsibility for determining needs, but the nurse informs and has current evidence and skills to impart.

(c) Patient centred – The nurse works alongside the patient, negotiating the role of the nurse as applicable to the situation and to individual patient needs. Within this model, there is the possibility for a therapeutic relationship to develop and for the nurse and patient to 'know' each other as people.

(d) Therapeutic relationship – Therapeutic relationship requires the nurse to respect and have genuine interest in the person, to show emotional warmth, tolerance and non-judgemental acceptance of the patient. It also calls for the practitioner to use 'self' in nursing interactions, whilst maintaining awareness of their limitations and adherence to ethical codes. The patient plays a part in a therapeutic relationship by trusting and co-operating with the intervention and being motivated to understand the treatment/care.

4   What is meant by the term 'emotional labour'.

The term emotional labour indicates the emotional work done as part of a job and is governed by 'feeling rules' set by the employer. These unarticulated rules of social interactions indicate how deeply we should feel and for how long. Expectations for emotional labour tend to be linked to female-dominated work roles.

5   What do the letters PDSA stand for in the service improvement cycle?

In the service improvement cycle, the letters PDSA stand for:

Plan / **D**o / **S**tudy / **A**ct.

6 **How might a multidisciplinary team that could be described as 'committed' (Bruce, 1980) show that they are working interprofessionally?**

A multidisciplinary team described as 'committed' (Bruce, 1980) could show that they are working interprofessionally by investing time and energy into their teamwork.

Chapter 10

1 **Give four teaching methods that could help to integrate theory and practice.**

Teaching methods that could help to integrate theory and practice are:

- problem-based learning (can be based around one patient case, a patient problem, a clinical skill, an ethical or professional dilemma)
- team teaching involving lecturers and clinical staff
- accrediting work-based learning
- recording and reviewing role-play communications
- well-designed interactive e-learning with sufficient computer access time and skills (Atack and Rankin, 2002)
- access to evidence-based information within academic and practical settings
- clinical skills laboratories that allow the simulation of health care environments
- action learning sets
- patient teaching
- tutorials and discussion groups
- workshops
- personal development plans.

2 **Why are academic and service partnerships being encouraged?**

Academic and service partnerships are being encouraged because they:

- enable sharing good practice and innovation nationally
- assist statutory bodies to maintain their obligations to protect the public
- provide evidence on the quality of higher education in health care provision
- ensure education is of a high quality for future employees.

3 **What reasons could a learning organisation give for encouraging the continuous professional development of its employees?**

The reasons that a learning organisation could give for encouraging the continuous professional development of its employees are:

- education and CPD activities impact on practitioners' ability to deliver health services as part of a flexible competent workforce (DoH, 1997b).
- CPD enhances knowledge and skills
- there is a positive correlation between professional development and staff satisfaction, staff retention and quality patient care
- ability to access to lifelong learning activities is aligned to recruitment and retention in the clinical setting.

4 **What is a training needs analysis?**

A Training Needs Analysis (TNA) informs decision-making and is part of an education strategy. A training needs analysis gives a baseline set of data for what training has been undertaken and what additional training is required; it identifies priorities and gives feedback as to the effectiveness of previous decisions.

5 **What activities may a nurse teacher undertake within a clinical setting?**

The activities that a nurse teacher may undertake within a clinical setting are:

- acting as a link lecturer, talking with staff and students
- supporting mentor and practice teacher development
- active clinical role
- professional and practice development
- contributing to practice research
- involvement in action learning sets
- supporting clinical leadership development.

6 **List at least four community-of-practice processes that can occur in nursing teams.**

Community of practice processes that can occur in nursing teams are:

- fostering a 'facilitative culture'
- development of situated leadership

- encouraging lifelong learning and continuous professional development
- utilising prioritisation frameworks
- implementing situated changes

- combining care activities
- sustaining communal memory
- reducing dissonance and conflict
- making personal learning explicit.

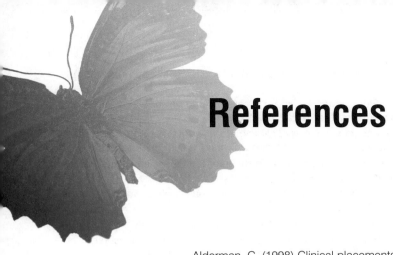

References

Alderman, C. (1998) Clinical placements. *Nursing Standard*, **12**(40), 22–24.

Alderson, J. and Wall, D. (1993) Does washback exist? *Applied Linguistics*, **14**(2), 115–129.

Allen, D. (2000) Negotiating the role of expert carers on an adult hospital ward. *Sociology of Health and Illness*, **22**(2), 149–171.

Andre, K. (2000) Grading student clinical practice performance: the Australian perspective. *Nurse Education Today*, **20**(8), 672–679.

Andrews, M. and Chilton, F. (2000) Student and mentor perceptions of mentor effectiveness. *Nurse Education Today*, **20**(7), 555–562.

Andrews, M. and Roberts, D. (2003) Supporting student nurses learning in and through practice: the role of the clinical guide. *Nurse Education Today*, **23**(7), 474–481.

Armstrong, P. and Armstrong, H. (1996) *Wasting away. The undermining of Canadian health care*. Oxford University Press, Toronto.

Atack, L. and Rankin, J. (2002) A descriptive study of registered nurses' experiences with web-based learning. *Journal of Advanced Nursing,* **40**(4), 457–465.

Audit Commission (2001) *Hidden Talents: education, training and development for health care staff in NHS Trusts*. Audit Commission National Report, London.

Bailey, D. (2005) Using an action research approach to involving service users in the assessment of professional competence. *European Journal of Social Work*, **8**(2), 165–179.

Bakker, A., Le Blanc, P., Schaufeli, W. (2005) Burnout contagion among intensive care nurses. *Journal of Advanced Nursing*, **51**(3), 276–287.

Barnett, R. (1997) *Higher Education: a critical business*. SRHE/Open University Press, Milton Keynes.

Barr, H., Hammick, M., Koppel, I. and Reeves, S. (1999) Evaluating interprofessional education: two systematic reviews for health and social care. *British Educational Research Journal*, **25**(4), 533–544.

Barrett, H. (2002) Directions in Electronic Portfolio Development. www.electronicportfolios.com

Batalden, P. and Stoltz, P. (1993) A framework for continuing improvement of health care: building and applying professional and improvement knowledge to test change in daily work. *The Joint Commission Journal on Quality Improvement*, **19**(10), 432–452.

Baxter Magolda, M. (1992) *Knowing and reasoning in college students: Gender-related patterns in students' intellectual development*. Jossey Bass, San Francisco.

Bechtel, G., Davidhizar, R. and Bradshaw, M. (1999) Problem-based learning in a competency-based world. *Nurse Education Today*, **19**(3), 182–187.

Bell, A., Horsfall, J. and Goodin, W. (1998) The mental health nursing clinical confidence scale: a tool for measuring undergraduate learning on mental health clinical placements. *Australian and New Zealand Journal of Mental Health*, **7**(4), 184–190.

Benner, P. (1984) *From Novice to Expert: Excellence and power in clinical nursing practice*. Addison-Wesley, Menlo Park, California.

Biggs, J. (2003) *Teaching for Quality Learning at University*, 2nd edn. The Society for Research into Higher Education and Open University Press, Buckingham.

Billett, S. (2001) Learning through working life: interdependencies at work. *Studies in Continuing Education*, **23**(1), 19–35.

Bolton, S. (2001) Changing faces: nurses as emotional jugglers. *Sociology of Health and Illness*, **23**(1), 85–100.

Borton, T. (1970) *Reach, Touch and Teach*. McGraw-Hill, New York.

Boud, D. and Walker, D. (1998) Promoting reflection in professional courses: the challenge of context. *Studies in Higher Education*, **23**(2), 191–206.

Bowers, B., Lauring, C. and Jacobsen, N. (2001) How nurses manage time and work in long-term care. *Journal of Advanced Nursing*, **33**(4), 484–491.

Boyd, E. and Fales, A. (1983) Reflective learning: key to learning from experience. *Journal of Humanistic Psychology*, **23**(2), 99–117.

Bruce, N. (1980) *Teamwork for Preventative Care*. John Wiley and Sons. Research Studies Press, Chichester.

Burgoyne, J. (1994) Introduction: established and emergent learning company concepts and practices. In: *Towards the Learning Company. Concepts and Practices* (ed. Burgoyne, J., Pedler, M. and Boydell, T.). McGraw-Hill Book Company, London, pp. 1–8.

Burke, L. and Harris, D. (2000) Education purchasers' views of nursing as an all graduate profession. *Nurse Education Today*, **20**(8), 620–628.

Burke, L. and Smith, P. (2000) Developing an audit tool for health promotion learning opportunities in clinical placements. *Nurse Education Today*, **20**(6), 475–484.

Burkitt, I., Husband, C., MacKenzie, J. and Tom, A. (2000) *Clinical Judgement and Nurse Education: Nursing Identities and Communities of Practice. Final Report*. University of Bradford and English National Board for Nursing, Midwifery and Health Visiting, London.

Butterworth, T., Carson, J., White, E., Jeacock, J., Clements, A. and Bishop, V. (1997) *Clinical Supervision and Mentorship: It's good to talk: An evaluation study in England and Scotland*. University of Manchester, Department of Nursing and Midwifery, Manchester.

CAIPE (1997) *Interprofessional Education – a definition*. Centre for the Advancement of Interprofessional Education, London.

Callaghan, M. (2003) Nursing morale: what is it like and why? *Journal of Advanced Nursing*, **42**(1), 82–89.

Candela, L., Dalley, K. and Benzel-Lindley, J. (2006) A case for learning-centered curricula. *Journal of Nursing Education*, **45**(2), 59–66.

Carper, B. (1978) Fundamental ways of knowing in nursing. *Advances in Nursing Science*, **1**(1), 13–23.

Castro, B., Eshleman, J. and Shearer, R. (1999) Using humor to reduce stress and improve relationships. *Seminars for Nurse Managers*, **7**(2), 90–92.

Challis, M. (1993) *Introducing APEL*. Routledge, London.

Channell, W. (2002) Helping students to learn in the clinical environment. *Nursing Times*, **98**(39), 34–35.

Chesser-Smyth, P. (2005) The lived experiences of general student nurses on their first clinical placement: a phenomenological study. *Nurse Education in Practice*, **5**(6), 320–327.

Clark, R. and Ivanic, R. (1997) *Politics of Writing*. Routledge, London.

Coffield, F., Moseley, D., Hall, E. and Ecclestone, K. (2004) *Learning Styles and Pedagogy in Post-16 Learning: A systematic and critical review*. Learning Skills Research Council, London.

Cole, M., John-Steiner, S., Scribner, E. and Souberman, E. (eds) (1978) *L. S. Vygotsky Mind in Society: The development of higher psychological processes*. Harvard University Press, Cambridge, MA.

Connexions (2003) *Learning and Young People*. Department for Education and Skills, Sheffield, p.12.

Connor, M. (2004) The practical discourse in philosophy and nursing: an exploration of linkages and shifts in the evolution of praxis. *Nursing Philosophy*, **5**(1), 54–66.

Cope, P., Cuthbertson, P. and Stoddart B. (2000) Situated learning in the practice placement. *Journal of Advanced Nursing*, **31**(4), 850–856.

Corlett, J. (2000) The perceptions of nurse teachers, student nurses and preceptors of the theory–practice gap in nurse education. *Nurse Education Today*, **20**(6), 499–505.

Costello, J. and Horne, M. (2001) Patients as teachers? An evaluative study of patients' involvement in classroom teaching. *Nurse Education in Practice*, **1**(2), 94–102.

Covey, S. (1999) *The Seven Habits of Highly Effective People*. Simon & Schuster, London.

Cowan, J. (1998) *On Becoming an Innovative University Teacher: Reflection in action*. Society for Research into Higher Education and Open University Press, Buckingham.

Cowan, J. (2002) *Developing Skills, Abilities or Capabilities: Implications for educational developers*. Staff and Educational Developers Association. Routledge Falmer, London, 1.2, pp.1–4.1.2.

Cox, J.L., Holden, J.M. and Sagovsky, R. (1987) Detection of postnatal depression: development of the Edinburgh Postnatal Depression Scale. *British Journal of Psychiatry*, **150**, 782–786.

Crawford, M. and Kiger, A. (1998) Development through self-assessment strategies used during clinical nursing placements. *Journal of Advanced Nursing*, **27**(1), 157–164.

Crooks, D., Carpio, B., Brown, B., Black, M., O'Mara, L. and Noesgaard, C. (2005) Development of professional confidence by post diploma baccalaureate nursing students. *Nurse Education in Practice*, **5**(6), 360–367.

Crotty, M. (1993) Clinical role activities of nurse teachers in Project 2000 programmes. *Journal of Advanced Nursing*, **18**, 460–464.

Cushen, N. and Wigens, L. (2000) A staff support mechanism: the transformational partnership. *British Journal of Nursing*, **19**(16), 1074–1078.

Darling, L. (1984). What do nurses want in a mentor? *Journal of Nursing Administration*, **14**(10), 42–44.

Davies, C. (1995) *Gender and the Professional Predicament in Nursing*. Open University Press, Buckingham.

DeFillippi, R. (2001) Introduction: Project-based learning, reflective practices and learning outcomes. *Management Learning*, **32**(1), 5–10.

Department of Health (1997) *Education and Training Plan Guidance*. HMSO, London.

Department of Health (1999) *Making a Difference: Strengthening the nursing, midwifery and health visiting contribution to health and health care*. HMSO, London.

Department of Health (2000a) *Making a Difference in Primary Care: the challenge for nurses, midwives and health visitors*. Case Studies from NHS Regional Conferences. HMSO, London.

Department of Health (2000b) *Improving Working Lives*. Standard (22356). HMSO, London.

Department of Health (2000c) *The NHS Plan – A plan for investment. A plan for reform*. HMSO, London.

Department of Health (2002) *Funding Learning and Development for the Health care Workforce. Consultation on the review of contract benchmarking for NHS funded education and training*. HMSO, London.

Department of Health (2003) *Streamlining Quality Assurance in Health Care Education. Purpose and Action*. HMSO, London.

Department of Health (2004) *The NHS Knowledge and Skills Framework (NHSKSF) and Development Review Process*. Department of Health, Crown Publishers, London.

Dewey, J. (1938) *Experience and Education*. Collier, New York.

Dilbert, C. and Goldenberg, D. (1995). Preceptor's perceptions of benefits, rewards, supports and commitment to the preceptor role. *Journal of Advanced Nursing*, **21** (6), 1144–1151.

Dowswell, T., Hewison, J. and Hinds, M. (1998) Motivational forces affecting participation in post-registration degree courses and effects on home and work life: a qualitative study. *Journal of Advanced Nursing*, **28**(6), 1326–1333.

Dreier, O. (1996) Re-searching psychotherapeutic practice. In: *Understanding Practice: Perspectives on activity and context* (ed. Chaiklin, S. and Lave, J.). Cambridge University Press, Cambridge, Chapter 4, pp. 104–124.

Dreyfus, H. and Dreyfus, S. (1979) *What Computers Can't Do – The limits of artificial intelligence*. The Free Press, New York.

Duffy, K. (2004) *Failing Students*. NMC, London.

Dunn, R. (2003) The Dunn and Dunn learning style model and its theoretical cornerstone. In: *Synthesis of the Dunn and Dunn Learning Styles Model Research: Who, what, when, where and so what – the Dunn and Dunn learning styles model and its theoretical cornerstone* (ed. Dunn, R. and Griggs, S.). St John's University, New York, pp. 1–6.

Dunn, S. and Hansford, B. (1997) Undergraduate nursing students' perceptions of their clinical learning environment. *Journal of Advanced Nursing*, **25**(6), 1299–1306.

East Somerset NHS Trust (2000) *Clinical Supervision: Theoretical and practical approaches to the supervision of clinical practice*. East Somerset NHS Trust, Yeovil, Somerset.

Ebright, P., Urden Patterson, E. and Chalko, B. (2004) Themes surrounding novice nurse near-miss and adverse-event situations. *Journal of Nursing Administration*, **34**(11), 531–538.

Ecclestone, K. (1996) *How to Assess the Vocational Curriculum*. Kogan Page, London.

Edmond, C. (2001) A new paradigm for practice education. *Nurse Education Today*, **21**(4), 251–259.

Elkan, R. and Robinson, J. (1993) Project 2000: the gap between theory and practice. *Nurse Education Today*, **13**(4), 295–298.

Endacott, R., Gray, M., Jasper, M., McMullan, M., Miller, C., Scholes, J. and Webb, C. (2004) Using portfolios in the assessment of learning and competence: the impact of four models. *Nurse Education in Practice*, **4**(4), 250–257.

Engestrom, Y. (1994) *Training for Change: New approach to instruction and learning in working life*. International Labour Office, Geneva.

English, F. (1975) The three-cornered contract. *Transactional Analysis*, **5**(4), 383–384.

English National Board (1994) *Creating Lifelong Learners: Partnership for care*. London, ENB.

English National Board for Nursing, Midwifery and Health Visiting and the Department of Health (2001) *Placements in Focus: Developments in multiprofessional education: Guidance for education in practice for health care professionals*. ENB, London.

Eraut, M. (1994) *Developing Professional Knowledge and Competence* (4th edn., 1999) Falmer Press, Lewes.

Eraut, M. (2000a) The dangers in managing with an inadequate view of knowledge. A paper presented to the Third International Conference of Sociocultural Psychology – Turning Knowledge Management Upside Down. July, Brazil.

Eraut, M. (2000b) Non-formal learning and tacit knowledge in professional work. *British Journal of Educational Psychology*, **70**(1), 113–136.

Eraut, M., Alderton, J., Cole, G. and Senker, P. (1998) Learning from other people at work. In: *Learning at Work* (ed. Coffield, F.). The Policy Press, Bristol.

Farrell, G. (2001) From tall poppies to squashed weeds: why don't nurses pull together more? *Journal of Advanced Nursing*, **35**(1), 26–33.

Faugier, J. and Butterworth, T. (1992) *Clinical Supervision and Mentorship in Nursing*. Chapman and Hall, London.

Feldman, D. (1999). Toxic mentors or toxic protégés? A critical re-examination of dysfunctional mentoring. *Human Resource Management Review*, **9**(3), 247–278.

Ferguson, L. (1996) Preceptors enhance students' self-confidence. *Nursing Connections*, **9**(1) 49–61.

Field, D. (2004) Moving from novice to expert – the value of learning in clinical practice: a literature review. *Nurse Education Today*, **24**(7), 560–565.

Fish, D. and Coles, C. (eds.) (1998) *Developing Professional Judgement in Health Care: Learning through the critical appreciation of practice*. Butterworth Heinemann, Oxford.

Fisher, M., Walsh, A. and Crouch, S. (2005) *Uncovering Skills for Practice*. Nelson Thornes, Cheltenham.

Flagler, S., Lopez-Powers, S. and Spitzer, A. (1988) Clinical teaching is more than evaluation alone! *Journal of Nurse Education*, **27**(8), 342–348.

Flanagan, J. (1954) The critical incident technique. *Psychological Bulletin*, **51**(4), 327–358.

Foucault, M. (1972) *The Archaeology of Knowledge*. Routledge, London.

Fox, R., Mazmanaian, P. and Putnam, R. (1989) *Changing and Learning in the Lives of Physicians*. Praeger, New York.

Freeth, D. and Reeves, S. (2004) Learning to work together: using presage, process, and product (3P) model to highlight decisions and possibilities. *Journal of Interprofesssional Care*, **18**(1), 43–56.

Gagné, R. (1985) *The Conditions of Learning and the Theory of Instruction*. Holt, Reinhart and Wilson, New York.

Gaines, C., Jenkins, S. and Ashe, W. (2005) Empowering nursing faculty and students for community service. *Journal of Nursing Education*, **44**(11), 522–525.

Gee, J. (2004) *Situated Language and Learning: A critique of traditional schooling*. Routledge, London.

Gerrish, K. (2000) Still fumbling along? A comparative study of the newly qualified nurse's perception of the transition from student to qualified nurse. *Journal of Advanced Nursing*, **32**(2), 473–480.

Gibbs, G. (1988) *Learning by Doing: A guide to teaching and learning methods*. Oxford Further Education Unit, Oxford.

Goleman, D. (1995) *Emotional Intelligence*. Bantam Books, New York.

Goodman, J. (1989) Reflection and teacher education: a case study and theoretical analysis. *Interchange*, **15**(3), 9–26.

Gopee, N. (2002) Human and social capital as facilitators of lifelong learning initiated through informal facilitators of learning through work based contacts with other health care professionals. *Nurse Education Today*, **22**(8), 608–616.

Gough, P. (2001) Changing culture and deprofessionalisation. *Nursing Management*, **7**(9), 8–9.

Grant, A. (2000) Clinical supervision and organisational power: a qualitative study. *Health and Learning Disabilities Care*, **3**(12), 398–401.

Greenhalgh, T. and Worrall, J. (1997) From EBM to CSM: the evolution of context sensitive medicine. *Journal of Evaluation in Clinical Practice*, **3**(2), 105–108.

Hall, V. and Hart, A. (2004) The use of imagination in professional education to enable learning about disadvantaged clients. *Learning in Health and Social Care*, **3**(4), 190–202.

Hammick, M. (1998) Interprofessional education: concept, theory and application. *Journal of Interprofessional Care*, **12**(3), 323–332.

Hammick, M. (2000) Interprofessional education: evidence from the past to guide the future. *Medical Teacher*, **22**(5), 472–478.

Harrison, R., Reeve, F., Hanson, A. and Clarke, J. (2002) (eds.) *Supporting Lifelong Learning*. Vol. 1. Perspectives on Learning. Routledge Falmer, London.

Hart, G. and Rotem, A. (1995) The clinical learning environment: nurse perceptions of professional development in clinical practice. *Nurse Education Today*, **15**(1), 3–10.

Harvey, G., Loftus-Hills, A., Rycroft-Malone, J., Titchen, A., Kitson, A., McCormack, B. and Seers, K. (2002) Getting evidence into practice: the role and function of facilitation. *Journal of Advanced Nursing*, **37**(6), 577–588.

Hatton, N. and Smith, D. (1995) Reflection in teacher education – towards definition and implementation. *Teaching and Teacher Education*, **11**(1), 33–49.

Hawkins, P. and Shohet, R. (1989) *Supervision in the Helping Professions: An individual, group and organizational approach.* Open University Press, Milton Keynes.

Health Professions Council (2004) Continuing Professional Development – Consultation paper. HPC, London.

Health Professions Council (2005) *Continuing Professional Development – Key Decisions*. HPC, London

Heitlinger, A. (1999) Nurses and nursing: a comparative perspective. *Journal of Interprofessional Care*, **13**(2), 165–174.

Henderson, A., Winch, S. and Heel, A. (2006) Partner, learn, progress: a conceptual model for continuous clinical education. *Nurse Education Today*, **26**(2), 104–109.

Heron, J. (1989) *Six Category Intervention Analysis*. Human potential resource group, University of Surrey, Guildford.

Hewinson, A. (1999) Nurses' power in interaction with patients. *Journal of Advanced Nursing*, **21**(1), 75–82.

Higher Education National Academy (2006) *National Professional Standards Framework for Teaching and Supporting Learning in Higher Education*. HENA, London.

Hislop, S., Inglis, B. and Cope, P. (1996) Situated theory in practice: student views of theory–practice in Project 2000 programmes. *Journal of Advanced Nursing*, **23**(1), 171–177.

Hochschild, A. (1983) *The Managed Heart: commercialisation of human feeling*. University of California Press, Berkeley.

Honey, P. and Mumford, A. (1992) *The Manual of Learning Styles*. Peter Honey Publications, Maidenhead.

Hopkinson, J. (2002) The hidden benefit: the supportive function of the nursing handover for qualified nurses caring for dying people in hospital. *Journal of Clinical Nursing*, **11**(2), 168–175.

Houle, C. (1961) *The Inquiring Mind: A study of the adult who continues to learn*. University of Wisconsin Press, Madison. Updated edition (1988) Research Center for Continuing Professional and Higher Education, University of Oklahoma, McCarter Hall.

Howell, W. and Fleishman, E. (1982) (eds.) *Human Performance and Productivity.* Vol. 2. Information Processing and Decision Making. Erlbaum, Hillsdale, NJ.

Ioannides, A. (1999) The nurse teacher's clinical role now and in the future. *Nurse Education Today*, **19**(3), 207–214.

Jacobs-Kramer, M. and Chinn, P. (1988) Perspectives on knowing: a model of nursing. *Scholarly Inquiry for Nursing Practice*, **2**(2), 129–139.

James, N. (1992) Care = Organisation + physical labour + emotional labour. *Sociology of Health and Illness*, **14**(5), 488–509.

Jarvis, P. (1995) *Adult and Continuing Education: Theory and practice*. Routledge, London.

Jarvis, P. and Gibson, S. (1997) *The Teacher Practitioner in Nursing, Midwifery and Health Visiting*, 2nd edn. Stanley Thornes Publishers, Cheltenham.

Jasper, M. (1996) The portfolio workbook as a strategy for student centred learning. In: *Closing the Theory–Practice Gap* (ed. Rolfe, G.). Butterworth Heinemann, Oxford.

Jasper, M (2003) Beginning Reflective Practice. *Foundations in Nursing and Health Care. Nelson Thornes, Cheltenham.*

Jasper, M. and Fulton, J. (2005) Marking criteria for assessing practice-based portfolios at masters' level. *Nurse Education Today*, **25**(5), 377–389.

Jasper, M., Rolfe, G. and Chambers, N. (2000) *Critical Reflection for Nursing and the Helping Professions*. Macmillan, Basingstoke.

Johns, C. (1998) Opening the doors of perception. In: *Transforming Nursing Through Reflective Practice* (ed. Johns, C. and Freshwater, D.). Blackwell Science, Oxford.

Johns, C. (2000) *Becoming a Reflective Practitioner*. Blackwell Science, Oxford.

Johns, C. and Freshwater, D. (1998) *Transforming Nursing Through Reflective Practice*. Blackwell, Oxford.

Johnson, D. and Johnson, R. (1992) *Advanced Cooperative Learning*. Interaction, MN.

Kadushin, A. (1992) *Supervision in Social Work, 3rd. edn*. Columbia University Press, New York.

Kirkpatrick, D. (1975) *Techniques for Evaluating Training Programmes*. American Society for Training and Development, Alexandria, VA.

Kneale, P. (1997) The rise of the 'strategic student': how can we adapt to cope? In: *Facing Up to Radical Changes in Universities and Colleges* (ed. Armstrong, S., Thompson, G. and Brown, S.). Kogan Page/SEDA, London.

Knowles, M. (1986) *Using Learning Contracts*. Jossey-Bass, San Francisco, CA.

Knowles, M. (1990) *The Adult Learner – A neglected species*. Gulf Publishing, Houston.

Koh, L. (2002) Practice-based teaching and nurse education. *Nursing Standard*, **16**(19), 38–42.

Kolb, D. (1984a) *Experiential Learning: Experience as a source of learning development*. Prentice Hall, Englewood Cliffs, NJ.

Kolb, D. (1984b) *Experiential Learning as the Science of Learning and Development*. Prentice Hall, Englewood Cliffs, NJ.

Kramer, M. (1974) *Reality Shock: Why nurses leave nursing*. Mosby, St Louis, MO.

Kristiansen, M. and Bloch-Poulsen, J. (2004). Self-referentiality as a power mechanism: towards dialogic action research. *Action Research*, **2**(4), 371–388.

Kyrkjebø, J. and Hage, I. (2005) What we know and what they do: nursing students' experiences of improvement knowledge in clinical practice. *Nurse Education Today*, **25**, 167–175.

Lauder, W., Reynolds, W. and Angus, N. (1999) Transfer of knowledge and skills: some implications for nursing and nurse education. *Nurse Education Today*, **19**(6), 480–487.

Lauder, W., Sharkey, S. and Booth, S. (2003) A case study of transfer of learning in a family health nursing course for students in remote and rural areas. *Nurse Education in Practice*, **4**(1), 39–44.

Lave, J. and Wenger, E. (1991) *Situated Learning – Legitimate Peripheral Participation*. Cambridge University Press, Cambridge.

Lawler, L. (1991) *Behind the Screens: Nursing, somology, and the problem of the body*. Churchill Livingstone, Melbourne.

LeMay, A. (1999) Knowledge for dissemination and implementation. In: *Nursing Research: Dissemination and implementation* (ed. Mulhall, A. and LeMay, A). Churchill Livingstone, Edinburgh.

Levett-Jones, T. (2005) Continuing education for nurses: a necessity or a nicety? *Journal of Continuing Education in Nursing*, **36**(5), 229–233.

Lewin, K. (1942) Field theory and learning. In: *Field Theory in Social Science: Selected theoretical papers* (1951) (ed. Cartwright, D.). Social Science Paperbacks, London.

Lines, H and Ricketts, B. (1994) Learning to achieve transformation in health. In: *Towards the Learning Company: Concepts and practices* (ed. Burgoyne, J., Pedler, M. and Boydell, T.). McGraw-Hill Book Company, London, Chapter 13, 158–168.

Little, V. (1999) The meaning of learning in critical care nursing: a hermeneutic study. *Journal of Advanced Nursing*, **30**(3), 697–703.

Lloyd Jones, M., Walters, S. and Akehurst, R. (2001) The implications of contact with the mentor for pre-registration nursing and midwifery students. *Journal of Advanced Nursing*, **35**(2), 151–160.

Macdonald, R. and Savin-Baden, M. (2004) *Assessment in Problem-Based Learning*. LTSN Generic Centre Assessment Series, No.7. LTSN Generic Centre, York.

Mackereth, P. (1989) An investigation of the developmental influences on nurse's motivation for their continuing education. *Journal of Advanced Nursing*, **14**(9), 776–778.

MacKinnon, G., McAllister, D. and Anderson S. (2001) Introductory practice experience: an opportunity for early professionalisation. *American Journal of Pharmaceutical Education*, **65**(3), 247–253.

Maeve, M. (1998) Weaving a fabric of moral meaning: how nurses live with suffering and death. *Journal of Advanced Nursing*, **27**(6), 1136–1142.

Manley, K. and McCormack, B. (1997) *Exploring Expert Practice* (NUM65U). Royal College of Nursing, London.

Manley, K., Hardy, S., Titchen, A., Garbett, R. and McCormack, B (2005) *Changing Patients' Worlds Through Nursing Practice Expertise*. A Royal College of Nursing Research Report, 1998–2004. RCN, London.

Marinker, M. (1974) Medical education and human values. *Journal of the Royal College of General Practitioners*, **24**(144)**,** 445–62.

Marton, F. and Saljo, R. (1984) Approaches to learning. In: *The Experience of Learning* (ed. Marton, F., Hounsell, D. and Entwhistle, N.). Scottish Academic Press, Edinburgh.

Maslow, A. (1954) *Motivation and Personality*. Harper, New York.

Maslow, A. (1970) *Motivation and Personality*. Harper and Row, New York.

Matthews, J. and Candy, P. (1999) New dimensions in the dynamics of learning and knowledge. In: *Understanding Learning at Work* (ed. Boud, D. and Garrick, J.). Routledge, London, pp. 47–64.

Maudsley, G. and Strivens, J. (2000) Promoting professional knowledge, experiential learning and critical thinking for medical students. *Medical Education*, **34**(7), 535–544.

McAllister, M. (2003) Doing practice differently: solution-focused nursing. *Journal of Advanced Nursing*, **41**(6), 528–535.

McCormack, B., Kitson, A., Harvey, G., Rycroft-Malone J., Titchen, A. and Seers, K. (2002) Getting evidence into practice: the meaning of 'context'. *Journal of Advanced Nursing*, **38**(1), 94–104.

McGarry, J. and Thorn, N. (2004) How users and carers view their involvement in nurse education. *Nursing Times*, **100**(18), 36–39.

McGrath, J. and Rotchford, N. (1983) Time and behavior in organizations. In: *Research in Organizational Behavior* (ed. Cummings, L. and Staw, B.). JAI Press, Greenwich, Chapter 5, 57–101.

McMullan, M., Endacott, R., Gray, M., Jasper, M., Miller, C., Scholes, J. and Webb, C. (2003) Portfolios and assessment of competence: a review of the literature. *Journal of Advanced Nursing*, **41**(3), 283–294.

Melia, K. (1987) *Learning and Working: The occupational socialization of nurses*. London, Tavistock.

Menzies, I. (1960) *The Functioning of Social Systems as a Defence Against Anxiety: A report on a study of the nursing service of a general hospital*. Tavistock, London.

Miers, M. (2002) Nurse education in higher education: understanding cultural barriers to progress. *Nurse Education Today*, **22**(3), 212–219.

Mikkelsen Kyrkjebø, J. and Hage, I. (2005) What we know and what they do: nursing students' experiences of improvement knowledge in clinical practice. *Nurse Education Today*, **25**(3), 167–175.

Mohammed, M. (2004) Using statistical process control to improve the quality of health care. *Quality and Safety in Health Care*, **13**(4), 243–245.

Moon, J. (1999) *Reflection in Learning and Professional Development: Theory and Practice*. Kogan Page, London.

Morton-Cooper, A. and Palmer, A. (1993) *Mentoring and Preceptorship*. Blackwell Science, Oxford.

Moseley, L., Mead, D. and Moran, L. (2004) An empirically derived clinical placement evaluation tool: a 3-country study. *Nurse Education Today*, **24**(5), 350–356.

Mulhall, A. (2002) Nursing research and nursing practice: an exploration of two different cultures. *Intensive and Critical Care Nursing*, **18**(1), 48–55.

Myers, I. and McCaulley, M. (1998) *Manual: A guide to the development and use of the Myers-Briggs Type Indicator*. Consulting Psychologists Press, Palo Alto, CA.

Myrick, F. and Yonge, O. (2001) Creating a climate for critical thinking in the preceptorship experience. *Nurse Education Today*, **21**(6), 461–467.

NHS Executive (1995) *Clinical Supervision: A resource pack*. Department of Health, London.

Nicol, M. and Freeth, D. (1998) Assessment of clinical skills: a new approach to an old problem. *Nurse Education Today*, **18**(8), 601–609.

Nolan, J. (2001) A flexible approach to Methicillin-Resistant Staphylococcus Aureus (MRSA). *Nursing Times*, **97**(46), 57–58.

Nolan, M., Owen, R. and Nolan, J. (1995) Continuing professional education: identifying the characteristics of an effective system. *Journal of Advanced Nursing*, **21**(3), 551–560.

Nursing and Midwifery Council (2002) *Standards for the Preparation of Teachers of Nursing and Midwifery*. NMC, London.

Nursing and Midwifery Council (2004a) *Standards of Proficiency for Pre-registration Nursing Education*. NMC, London.

Nursing and Midwifery Council (2004b) *Midwives Rules and Standards*. NMC, London.

Nursing and Midwifery Council (2004c) *The PREP Handbook*. NMC, London.

Nursing and Midwifery Council (2005) *Consultation on a Standard to Support Learning and Assessment in Practice: Issues arising from the consultation*. NMC, London.

Nursing and Midwifery Council (2006) Standard to support learning and assessment in practice: Draft March 2006 version. NMC, London.

Oakshott, M. (1962) *Rationalism in Politics and Other Essays*. Methuen and Co., London.

Ohlen, J. and Segesten, K. (1998) The professional identity of the nurse: concept analysis and development. *Journal of Advanced Nursing*, **28**(4), 720–727.

Ohrling, K. and Hallberg, I. (2001a) Nurses' lived experience of being a preceptor. *Journal of Professional Nursing*, **16**(4), 228–239.

Ohrling, K. and Hallberg, I. (2001b) The meaning of preceptorship: nurses' lived experience of being a preceptor. *Journal of Advanced Nursing*, **33**(4), 530–554.

Oliver, R. and Endersby, C. (2000) *Teaching and Assessing Nurses: A handbook for preceptors*. Bailliere Tindall, London.

Open University (2001). *Assessing Practice in Nursing and Midwifery*. Open University Press, Milton Keynes.

Orland-Barak, L. and Wilhelem, D. (2005) Novices in clinical practice settings: student nurses' stories of learning the practice of nursing. *Journal of Advanced Nursing*, **21**(1), 75–82.

Palmer, A., Burns, S. and Bulam, C. (1994) *Reflective Practice in Nursing: The growth of the professional practitioner*. Blackwell Science, Oxford.

Palmer S., Harmer Cox, A., Callister, L., Johnsen, V. and Matsumura, G. (2005) Nursing education and service collaboration: making a difference in the clinical learning environment. *Journal of Continuing Education in Nursing*, **36**(6), 271–276.

Papp, I., Markkanen, M. and von Bonsdorff, M. (2003) Clinical environment as a learning environment: student nurses' perceptions concerning clinical learning experiences. *Nurse Education Today*, **23**(4), 262–268.

Pardoe, S. (2000) A question of attribution: the interdeterminacy of learning from experience. In: *Student Writing in Higher Education* (ed. Lea, M. and Stierer, B.). SRHE/ Open University Press, Milton Keynes, pp. 123–145.

Parsons, T. (1968) Professions. In: *International Encyclopaedia of the Social Sciences* (ed. Sills, D.). Macmillan, New York, xii, pp. 536–547.

Patel, V., Arocha, J. and Kayfman, D. (1999) Medical cognition. In: *Handbook of Applied Cognition* (ed. Durso, F.). Wiley, New York, pp. 663–693.

Paton, B. (2003) Unready-to-hand as adventure: knowing within the practice wisdom of nurse educators. Unpublished PhD Nursing thesis. University of Wellington, Victoria.

Pearce, R. (2003) *Profiles and Portfolios of Evidence*. Foundations in Nursing and Health Care. Nelson Thornes, Cheltenham.

Pearcey, P. and Elliott, B. (2004) Student impressions of clinical nursing. *Nurse Education Today*, **24**(5), 382–387.

Perry-Woodford, Z. and Whayman, K. (2005) Education in practice: a colorectal link-nurse programme. *British Journal of Nursing*, **14**(16), 862–866.

Peyton, J. (1998) The learning cycle. In: *Teaching and Learning in Medical Practice* (ed. Peyton, J.). Manticore, Rickmansworth, pp. 13–19.

Pfeil, M. (2003) Assessing the clinical skills performance of nursing students. *Journal of Child Health Care*, **7**(3), 191–206.

Phillips, A, (1994) Creating space in the learning company. In: *Towards the Learning Company: Concepts and practices* (ed. Burgoyne, J., Pedler, M. and Boydell, T.). McGraw-Hill Book Company, London, pp. 98–109.

Phillips, T., Schostak, J. and Tyler, J. (2000a) *Practice and Assessment: An evaluation of the assessment of practice at diploma, degree and postgraduate level in pre and post registration nursing and midwifery education*. English National Board for Nursing, Midwifery and Health Visiting, London.

Phillips, T., Schostak, J. and Tyler, J. (2000b) *Practice and Assessment in Nursing and Midwifery: Doing it for real (PandA project)*. English National Board, London.

Piaget, J. (1971) *Biology and Knowledge*. Edinburgh University Press, Edinburgh.

Pirrie, A., Wilson, V., Elsegood, J., Hall, J., Hamilton, S., Harden, R., Lee, D. and Stead, J. (1998) *Evaluating Multidisciplinary Education in Health Care*. Scottish Council for Research Education, Edinburgh.

Playle, P. and Mullarkey, K. (1998) Parallel process in clinical supervision: enhancing learning and providing support. *Nurse Education Today, 18(7), 558–566.*

Polanyi, M. (1951) *The Logic of Liberty.* Routledge and Kegan Paul, London.

Price, B. (2004) Encouraging reflection and critical thinking in practice. *Nursing Standard*, **18**(47), 46–52.

Priest, H. (1999) Novice and expert perceptions of psychological care and the development of psychological caregiving abilities. *Nurse Education Today*, **19**(7), 556–563.

Proctor, B. (1987) Supervision: A co-operative exercise in accountability. In: *Enabling and Ensuring: Supervision in practice* (ed. Marken, M. and Payne, M.). National Youth Bureau, Leicester.

Quality Assurance Agency for Higher Education (2001) *Code of Practice for the Assurance of Academic Quality and Standards in Higher Education*. Section 9: Placement Learning. QAAHE, Gloucester.

Quinn, F. (1995) *The Principles and Practice of Nurse Education*. Chapman and Hall, Cheltenham, Chapter 11.

Ramsden, P. (1992) *Learning to Teach in Higher Education*. Routledge, London.

Randle, J. (2003) Changes in self-esteem during a 3-year pre-registration Diploma in Higher Education (Nursing) programme. *Journal of Clinical Nursing*, **12**(1), 142–143.

Richardson, B. (1999) Professional development: 2 Professional knowledge and situated learning in the workplace. *Physiotherapy*, **85**(9), 467–474.

Robinson, A., Murrell, T., Hickey, G., Clinton, M. and Tingle A. (2003) *A Tale of Two Courses: Comparing careers and competencies of nurses prepared via a three-year degree and three-year diploma courses*. Kings College, Nursing Research Unit, London.

Rogers C. (1967) The interpersonal relationships in the facilitation of learning. In: *Humanizing Education* (ed. Leeper, R). Association for Supervision and Curriculum Development, Alexandria VA.

Rogoff, B. (1990) *Apprenticeship in Thinking*. Oxford University Press, New York and Oxford.

Rolfe, G. (1993) Closing the theory-practice gap: a model of nursing praxis. *Journal of Clinical Nursing*, **2**(3), 173–177.

Rolfe, G. (2006) Nursing praxis and the science of the unique. *Nursing Science Quarterly*, **19**(1), 39–43.

Royal College of Nursing (2002a) *Helping Students Get the Best from Their Practice Placements: a Royal College of Nursing toolkit*. RCN, London.

Royal College of Nursing (2002b) Knowledge Utilisation: Practice Epistemology and Transformation in Practice. RCN Practice Development Institute Presentation to the Knowledge Utilisation Conference. St Catherine's College, Oxford.

Royal College of Nursing (2003) *The Future Nurse*. RCN Policy Unit, London.

Royal College of Nursing (2004) *The Future Nurse: The future for nurse education: a discussion paper*. RCN, London.

Ryan, J. (2003) Continuous professional development along the continuum of lifelong learning. *Nurse Education Today*, **23**(7), 498–508.

Sarup, M. (1996) *Identity, Culture and the Postmodern World*. Edinburgh University Press, Edinburgh.

Saunders, L. (1998) Managing delegation: a field study of a systematic approach to delegation in out-patient physiotherapy. *Physiotherapy*, **84**(11), 547–555.

Savin-Baden, M. (2000) *Problem-based Learning in Higher Education: Untold stories*. Open University Press, Buckingham.

Scanlon, J. and Chernomas, W. (1997) Developing the reflective teacher. *Journal of Advanced Nursing*, **25**(6), 1138–1143.

Scheffer, B. and Rubenfeld, M. (2000). A consensus statement on critical thinking in nursing. *Journal of Nursing Education*, **39**(8), 352–362.

Scholes, J., Webb, C., Gray, M., Endacott, R., Miller, C., Jasper, M. and McMullan, M. (2004). Making portfolios work in practice. *Journal of Advanced Nursing*, **46**(6), 595–603.

Schön, D. (1983) *The Reflective Practitioner: How professionals think in action*. Basic Books, New York.

Schuler, R. and Jackson, S. (1986) Managing Stress through PHRM practices: An uncertainty interpretation. In: *Research in Personnel and Human Resource Management,* Vol. 4. (ed. Rowland, R. and Ferris, G.). JAI Press, Greenwich, CT, pp. 183–224.

Shiu, A. (1998) Work and family role juggling and mood states of Hong Kong public health nurses with children. *Journal of Advanced Nursing*, **28**(1), 203–211.

Simons, H. and Parry-Crooke, G, (2001) *We All Thrive on Praise: The Certificate in Teaching for Medicine and Dentistry*. Independent External Evaluation. Kent, Surrey and Sussex Deanery.

Skinner, B. (1953) *Science and Human Behavior*. The Free Press, New York.

Slevin, O. and Buckenham, M. (1992) Project 2000: The teachers speak. *Innovations in the Nursing Curriculum*. Campion Press, Edinburgh.

Sloan, G. (2005) Clinical supervision: beginning the supervisory relationship. *British Journal of Nursing*, **14**(17), 918–923.

Sloan, G. and Watson, H. (2001) John Heron's six-category intervention analysis: towards understanding interpersonal relations and progressing the delivery of clinical supervision for mental health nursing in the United Kingdom. *Journal of Advanced Nursing*, **26**(2), 206–214.

Smith, J. and Topping, A. (2001) Unpacking the 'value added' impact of continuing professional education: a multi-method case study approach. *Nurse Education Today*, **21**(5), 341–349.

Smith, P. (1992) *The Emotional Labour of Nursing: How nurses care*. Macmillan, London.

Snelgrove, S. and Hughes, D. (2000) Interprofessional relations between doctors and nurses: perspectives from South Wales. *Journal of Advanced Nursing*, **31**(3), 661–667.

Spouse, J. (2001) Bridging theory and practice in the supervisory relationship: a sociocultural perspective. *Journal of Advanced Nursing*, **33**(4), 512–522.

Spouse, J. (2003) *Professional Learning in Nursing*. Blackwell, Oxford.

Staib, S. (2003). Teaching and measuring critical thinking. *Journal of Nursing Education*, **42**(11), 498–508.

Steinaker, N. and Bell, R (1979) *The Experiential Taxonomy: A new approach to teaching and learning*. Academic Press, New York.

Stephenson, J. (1992) Capability and quality in higher education. In: *Quality in Learning: A capability approach in higher education* (ed. Stephenson, J. and Weil, S.). Kogan Page, London.

Stephenson, K., Peloquin, S., Richmond, S., Hinman, M. and Christiansen, C. (2002) Changing educational paradigms to prepare health professionals for the 21st century. *Education for Health*, **15**(1), 37–49.

Stevens, K. and Ledbetter, C. (2000) Basics of evidence based practice. Part 1: The nature of evidence. *Seminars in Perioperative Nursing*, **9**(3), 91–97.

Stoltenberg, C. D. and Delworth, U. (1987) *Supervising Counsellors and Therapists*. Jossey-Bass, San Francisco, CA.

Stordeur, S., D'Hoore, W. and Vandenberghe, C. (2001) Leadership, organizational stress, and emotional exhaustion among hospital nursing staff. *Journal of Advanced Nursing*, **35**(4), 533–542.

Suikkala, A. and. Leino-Kilpi, H. (2005) Nursing student–patient relationship: experiences of students and patients. *Nurse Education Today*, **25**(5), 344–354.

Tennant, M. (2005) *Psychology and Adult Learning*, 3rd edn. Routledge, London.

Thompson, C., McCaughan, D., Cullum, N., Shelden, T., Mulhall, A. and Thompson, D. (2001) Research information in nurses' clinical decision-making: What is useful? *Journal of Advanced Nursing*, **36**(3), 376–388.

Thorndike, E. (1913) The psychology of learning. *Educational Psychology 2*, Teachers' College Columbia University, New York.

Thorpe, K. (2004) Reflective learning journals: from concept to practice. *Reflective Practice*, **5**(3), 1–18.

Titchen, A. (2000) Professional craft knowledge in patient-centred nursing and facilitation of its development. Unpublished PhD Thesis. University of Oxford, Oxford.

Titmus, C. (1999) Concepts and practices of education and adult education: obstacles to lifelong education and lifelong learning. *International Journal of Lifelong Education*, **18**(3), 343–354.

Tiwari, A. and Tang, C. (2003) From process to outcome: the effect of portfolio assessment on student learning. *Nurse Education Today*, **23**(4), 269–277.

Tryssenar, J. and Perkins, J. (2001) From student to therapist: exploring the first year of practice. *American Journal of Occupational Therapy*, **55**(1), 19–27.

Tuckman, B. and Jensen, M. (1977). Stages of small group development revisited. *Group and Organization Studies*, **2**(4), 419–427.

Tye, C. and Ross, F. (2000) Blurring boundaries: professional perspectives of the ENP role in a major accident and emergency department. *Journal of Advanced Nursing*, **31**(5), 1089–1096.

United Kingdom Central Council for Nursing Midwifery and Health Visiting (1996) *Position Statement on Clinical Supervision for Nursing and Health Visiting*. UKCC London.

United Kingdom Central Council for Nursing, Midwifery and Health Visiting and Department of Health (1999) *Fitness for Practice*. UKCC, London.

Usher, R. and Soloman, N. (1999) Experiential learning and the shaping of subjectivity in the workplace. *Studies in the Education of Adults*, **31**(2), 155–163.

Wagner, F. (1957). Supervision of psychotherapy. *American Journal of Psychotherapy*, **11**(4), 759–768.

Wallace, B. (2003) Practical issues of student assessment. *Nursing Standard*, **17**(31), 33–36.

Walsh, M. and Wigens, L. (2003) *Introduction to Research*. Nelson Thornes, Cheltenham.

Wanless, D. (2004) *Securing Good Health for the Whole Population*. HM Treasury, London.

Weidman, J., Twale., D. and Stein, E. (2001) Socialisation of graduate and professional students in higher education. *ASHE-ERIC Higher Education Report*, **28**(3), Wiley Interscience, San Francisco.

Wenger, E. (1998) *Communities of Practice: Learning, meaning and identity*. Cambridge University Press, Cambridge.

Wenger, E. McDermott, R. and Snyder, W. (2002) *Cultivating Communities of Practice*. Harvard Business School Press, Boston.

Wigens, L. (1997) The conflict between 'new nursing' and 'scientific management' as perceived by surgical nurses. *Journal of Advanced Nursing*, **25**(6), 1116–1122.

Wigens, L. (1998) Specialist practice and the professional project for nursing. *British Journal of Nursing*, **7**(5), 266–269.

Wigens, L. (1999) The impact of an English National Board breast care course [ENB NO9] on registered nurses' interprofessional collaboration. Conference Presentation: Breakthrough Breast Cancer Conference, London.

Wigens, L. (2004) A case study of registered (care of the adult) nurses' management of individual caring in multiple demand settings, and the influence on this of situated learning. Unpublished PhD thesis. Norwich, University of East Anglia.

Wigens, L. (2005) Care in the multidisciplinary team. In: *Principles of Caring* (ed. McGee, P.). Nelson Thornes, Cheltenham.

Wigens, L. and Westwood, S. (2000) Issues surrounding educational preparation for intensive care nursing in the 21st century. *Intensive and Critical Care Nursing*, **16**(4), 221–227.

Wildman, S., Weale, A., Rodney, C. and Pritchard, J. (1999) The impact of higher education for post-registration nurses on their subsequent clinical practice: an exploration of students' views. *Journal of Advanced Nursing*, **29**(1), 246–253.

Williams, A. and Sibbald, B. (1999) Changing roles and identities in primary health care: exploring a culture of uncertainty. *Journal of Advanced Nursing*, **29**(3), 737–745.

Williams, P. (1998) Using theories of professional knowledge and reflective practice to influence educational change. *Medical Teacher*, **20**(1), 28–34.

Williamson, G. and Dodds, S. (1999) The effectiveness of a group approach to clinical supervision in reducing stress: a review of the literature. *Journal of Clinical Nursing*, **8**(4), 338–344.

Wilson, V. and Pirrie, A. (2000) *Multidisciplinary Teamworking: Beyond the barriers? A review of the issues*. Research Report No 96. Scottish Council for Research in Education, Edinburgh.

Wilson-Barnett, J., Butterworth, T., White, E., Twinn, S., Davies, S. and Riley, L. (1995) Clinical support and the Project 2000 nursing student: factors influencing this process. *Journal of Advanced Nursing*, **21**(6), 1152–1158.

Witz, A. (1992) *Professions and Patriarchy*. Routledge, London.

Wolff, A. and Rideout, E. (2001). The faculty role in problem-based learning. In: *Transforming Nursing Education through Problem-based Learning* (ed. Rideout, E). Jones and Bartlett, Sudbury, MA.

Wood, I. (1998) The ENB 199: an exploration of its effects on A & E nurses' practice. *Accident and Emergency Nursing*, **6**(4), 219–225.

Index